Delivering the Vision

Political rhetoric surrounding the role of information and knowledge in society in the twenty-first century is often thrown into sharp relief by the realities of practice. *Delivering the Vision* explores the way in which public service 'visions' have developed globally and how successful they have been in contributing to major social and economic change.

This edited text contains a range of case studies from the United Kingdom, the Republic of Ireland, Canada, the USA and Australia. Contributors focus both on those factors critical to success and on reasons for failure, but a common theme to emerge across all contributions is the requirement for a clear political vision, commitment and leadership if the shift from traditional forms of social and economic organisation to high-value, knowledge-intensive economies is to be safely negotiated. At the same time, individual case studies provide valuable blueprints for successful implementation of an ambitious public service change agenda.

Delivering the Vision is a practitioner-focused text, accessible and relevant to all those interested in the management and reform of public sector organisations. It is a companion volume to the editor's earlier text *Managing Information and Knowledge in the Public Sector* (Routledge 2000).

Eileen M. Milner is Principal Lecturer in Information Management at the University of North London.

Delivering the Vision

Public services for the information society and the knowledge economy

Edited by Eileen M. Milner

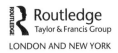
Routledge
Taylor & Francis Group

LONDON AND NEW YORK

First published 2002
by Routledge
2 Park Square, Milton Park, Abingdon, Oxon OX14 4RN

Simultaneously published in the USA and Canada
by Routledge
711 Third Avenue, New York, NY 10017

Routledge is an imprint of the Taylor & Francis Group an informa business

Typeset in Times New Roman by Exe Valley Dataset Ltd, Exeter

British Library Cataloguing in Publication Data
A catalogue record for this book is available from the British Library

Library of Congress Cataloging in Publication Data

Delivering the vision : public services for the information society and the knowledge
economy / edited by Eileen M. Milner.
    p. cm.
  Includes bibliographical references and index.
  1. Public administration–Information technology–Case studies. 2. Political
leadership–Case studies. 3. Internet in public administration–Case studies.
4. Information technology–Political aspects–Case studies. 5. Knowledge
management–Case studies. 6. Electronic government information–Case studies.
I. Milner, Eileen M., 1963–

JF525.A8 D43 2002
306.2–dc21   2001048185

ISBN 978-0-415-24155-7 (pbk)
ISBN 978-0-415-24154-0 (hbk)

This book is dedicated to Isabel Margaret Patricia Atkinson

Contents

Illustrations

Figures

Tables

Notes on contributors

Janet Caldow is director of IBM's Institute for Electronic Government based in Washington DC. The institute is a global leadership resource for governance, economic development, citizen services, technology, education and healthcare for the digital society. She serves on the Harvard Policy Group, the Congressional Management Foundation's Expert Panel on Congress Online, the World Bank and the e-communities task force.

Judith Dionysius is currently project director for the Customer Relationship Management Program at the National Roads and Motoring Association Member Services, Australia. Previously she was Customer Service Manager with Brisbane City Council, a position drawing upon her extensive career experience in information technology applications within government.

Mary Harney has been Tanaiste (deputy prime minister) of the Republic of Ireland since 1997, the first woman to have held this position. In addition she is Minister for Enterprise, Employment and Trade. A member of the Irish Parliament since 1981,she became leader of her political party, the Progressive Democrats, in 1995.

Paul Joyce is a professor based at Nottingham Trent University. His latest books include *Strategic Management for the Public Services* (Open University Press 1999), *Strategy in the Public Sector: A Guide to Effective Change Management* (Wiley 2000) and (with Adrian Woods) *Strategic Management* (Kogan Page 2001). He has advised the UK Cabinet Office on performance management in regulatory services, carried out evaluation research on best value and social inclusion in local government, and researched strategic management, leadership and innovation.

Eileen M. Milner is Principal Lecturer in information management at the University of North London. Author of *Managing Information and Knowledge in the Public Sector* (Routledge 2000) she both teaches and researches in these areas. Research and consultancy activities have been undertaken on behalf of both the United Kingdom and other governments.

Dawn Nicholson-O'Brien is a senior visiting research fellow with the Canadian Centre for Management Development, where she specialises in knowledge creation and innovation within government. Within this role she is specifically addressing the area of innovation and connection within a Canadian context. She has served as an executive within a number of departments during a public service career of some 20 years. She is also currently pursuing doctoral studies.

Susan Pollonetsky is a senior advisor to the Canadian Treasury Board Secretariat based within its Corporate Renewal and Knowledge Management Office. In this role she has been active in promoting knowledge management and allied innovation across Canadian government.

Sue Vardon has been chief executive of Centrelink since its creation in 1997. Previously she had held chief executive officer posts within Community Services, Public Sector Reform and Correctional Services. She is a Fellow of the Australian Institute of Management and of the Institute of Public Administration, Australia becoming the president of the latter in 2000. She is also an adjunct professor of the Institute of Governance at the University of Canberra.

Preface

Mathematical purists heralded the commencement of the twenty-first century as being the dawn of the year 2001, if this were so, then in terms of the information society at least, it was a dawn clouded by the complexities and anxieties arising from the presidential election 'outcome' in the United States. The world's last global superpower found itself the subject of internal wrangling both political and legal, and external incredulity that the democratic process could have unravelled to such an extent that chaos did indeed reign for a period of several weeks. The cause of all of this uncertainty was the perceived and actual unreliability of electoral data and the apparent lack of robustness in the methods for collecting and analysing it. As a case study in modern democracy it is, perhaps, a salutary reminder that the rhetoric surrounding the role of information in society can be thrown into somewhat stark relief by the realities of actual practice.

Consider too the term *knowledge economy*. It too is a phrase familiar to politicians, although what precisely they mean by it, beyond an aspiration to create greater employment in technology-based industries, is, more often than not, poorly articulated. However, if we take accepted definitions of knowledge as being something tacit, not normally articulated in a readily collectable form, but possessing some intrinsic value when extracted and analysed, then once more we can see the capacity for governments to be less than successful in this area of activity. So, for example, in April 2001 the United Kingdom undertook its census of the population, the first since 1991, and much heralded in respect of the advances anticipated from increased use of information and communications technologies. However, early analysis of the exercise, as reported widely in UK media, indicates that rather than improving the quantity and speed of information gathering and processing, providing key knowledge assets to feed into planning and policy formation processes, that the levels of citizen input achieved have been less than those achieved over 100 years ago. Instead of maximising the potential for extracting valuable knowledge assets, the process has, instead, proved to be successful in the key negative indicator areas of chaos creation and the engendering of public antipathy towards the process.

It was fortuitous perhaps that the commencement of the year 2001 provided such a rich context for the preparation of a text such as this. However, when developing a rationale for this edited text, the guiding principle was to focus upon drawing together a range of perspectives which would serve to illuminate the role of government and of public services more generally in delivering the much vaunted aspirations to reside in 'information societies' and 'knowledge economies'.

Rarely, as outlined in the two opening vignettes, can two terms have proved as universally popular with politicians of virtually every persuasion, on a truly global stage, yet with no clear articulation of what is actually meant by these words. It is important to ask, do they actually have any resonance with citizens' actual experience of life and key episodes within it? Or, are both the information society and the knowledge economy, simply catchy soundbites on which politicians hope to move forward their own rather more traditional agenda?

The philosophy underpinning all the contributions to this work is that society has changed and continues to change, and that a key driver in this process has been the opportunities afforded for enhancement of communication and connectivity facilitated by developments in information and communication technologies (ICTs). Technological developments have made possible a way of life where assumptions which less than a decade ago held true, around established concepts of space and time. For example, the notion of office hours only operation and of a fixed point of contact, continue to be challenged and expectations raised in respect of the possibilities for change. In reality this is where the critical challenges around realising the information society and knowledge economy actually reside. The challenge for public services is to maintain or perhaps refocus their very reasons for existing, to prove themselves to be relevant to citizens who are increasingly disengaged from the mainstream of the democratic process. Further, a key aspiration for public services, must also surely be that they help to build a culture and climate where the promised returns of the information society and knowledge economy are a reality for a majority rather than being the territory of a small elite.

Within what is generally termed *society*, the new attitudes and models of behaviour referred to above, are fast becoming the norm for a significant proportion of the population. However, there is, allied to this development, a danger that what might be termed a New Darwinism is beginning to emerge, where a process of natural selection is seeing high value, knowledge workers emerge, whose lives are reliant for support by a large tranche of service workers. Such developments leave exposed two distinctly vulnerable groups in society, the first, those who for reasons of socio-economic factors have traditionally been excluded from the education and development support available to the mainstream of society. However, the second group may be just as significant, it is made up of those who had previously provided the solid middle strata of society, who provided the bureaucracy and the systems which served to support organisations and wider society. Public service models extant across the globe provide a range of offerings aimed at both the many and at more targeted excluded strata. However, in many instances, they, like commercial sector organisations before them, have also been focusing upon divesting themselves of their own middle layers. There has been an emerging view that high value (value accruing from citizen perception and engagement primarily), effective public services will naturally evolve from the placing of emphasis upon information processing technologies and the efforts of key knowledge elites. The purpose of this text is to provide an evidence base upon which to assess how far, and with what degree of success, public services have moved towards adoption of this model and, where appropriate, to challenge its appropriateness.

The title of this text refers to the need for vision in respect of successful public service engagement with the concepts of the information society and the knowledge economy. The underpinning need for leadership, the foundations of an articulation of the vision element, permeates almost every contribution to the work. Indeed a pattern can be clearly delineated which sees the pivotal role which politicians play in setting a clear enabling agenda in respect of attaining the benefits of information and knowledge within a wider societal context. Such overt political leadership on these linked agenda, as evidenced in the Brisbane city council case study, the discussions by both Harney and Joyce in respect of the Republic of Ireland and in the analysis of Nicholson-O'Brien, demonstrate the critical role of early and ongoing input by senior level politicians when seeking to deliver a major public service change agenda. Leadership too must come from those charged with operationalising major realignment in public service structures and functions. Here the contributions by Vardon and Caldow provide consider-able insight into the challenges that such figures face when attempting to reconcile political aspirations with the realities of complex and legacy-based public service structures.

Critically then the theme of delivery is linked by all contributors to this work to that of vision. Leadership in itself is certainly essential but so too is having a mandate to actually enact the type and scale of change typically required. The benchmark of success in this area should not be the existence of well-drafted policy and strategy documents, but rather must focus upon what has actually been delivered in respect of changes to the way in which public services do business.

An additional theme, that of the need for ongoing revision, is considered by almost every contributor to this text – the common theme here being the imperative to acknowledge and be able to respond to changes in capacity and potential, as well as citizen expectation. Common characteristics across all areas of public service provision considered in this work, emerge from the sheer pressure for ongoing change that has become the norm within organisations across all sectors but which presents significant challenges for within this area. The dynamic created by achieving high levels of service enhancement, as discussed by Dionysius, serves to add a further pressure of both base level resourcing and management capacity to keep pace with the growing citizen enthusiasm for re-engineered public services.

In terms of structure, there are four main strands contained within this work, focusing on key areas of public policy and allied service development, these are:

1 By way of introduction, the chapters by Milner and Caldow consider critical challenges facing the public service community as they seek to position themselves to both enable and support, as well as deliver on aspects of, the information society and the knowledge economy. Caldow identifies seven milestones which, she argues, are critical, if governments are to move forward to release potential for both social and economic benefits to accrue to the widest possible interpretation of society. Milner's focus is on consideration of an underpinning agenda for change which she argues is generalisable across all public service applications.

2 Australia has become globally recognised as a key learning laboratory in respect of public service reform and it is appropriate here that two key expemplar sites should be put forward for consideration. Brisbane City Council and Centrelink represent two major case studies in service re-engineering, the scope and scale of which make them relevant to all of those with an interest in this area of development. In the case of both studies, the pivotal role of having political leadership and input from the outset is clearly articulated. So too are the challenges of keeping pace with the momentum of change which, once unleashed, forms an ongoing challenge to those seeking to manage emerging demands and technological possibilities, in a pragmatic and responsible manner.

3 Pollonetsky and Nicholson-O'Brien provide valuable perspective on the way in which people are key repositories of knowledge which can be usefully harnessed to leverage the perceived value and effectiveness of public services. Both contributors provide insights from the Canadian approach to harnessing public service employee and citizen input in a positive and change-focused manner. As with the Australian case studies, what is noticeable once more in these wide-ranging analyses of approaches adopted in Canada, has been the key requirement for leadership and political engagement to be evident throughout change processes.

4 The final substantive section takes a holistic view of one nation's approach to delivering on the challenges of the information society and the knowledge economy. The Republic of Ireland, the Deputy Prime Minister Mary Harney argues, has achieved economic success and wider societal inclusion, through the development of coherent and cohesive policies to

enable and support a climate for economic and social change. Further analysis of this view is provided by Joyce who, whilst considering the nation state as an entity, takes the opportunity to also bore down into more local level interpretations of Irish policy in this area. Joyce also questions the capacity of public services more generally to engage in the challenges of change required of them.

Thus, within this text the themes of vision, delivery and revision are discussed in relation, whenever possible, to the realities of the applied public service environment. Where case studies are provided, they have earned their place on the basis of being recognised as providing world class exemplars of practice in this area. The role of information and communications technologies as a key driver of change is, of course, discussed in almost every chapter. However, all contributors broadly concur that the key area of focus should be upon moving away from any sense of technologies providing solutions to public service challenges, but rather to consider their role as enablers of properly constructed rationale for service redesign within a wider framework of information and knowledge becoming key global currencies.

In terms of provenance, this text is, in terms of its contributors, a truly global analysis of policy and practice. However, it may be a matter of some conjecture as to why there is no specific use of the United Kingdom as a case study within this work. The response to such questions is not to detract in any way from the many innovative approaches to service redesign evident within the UK at the time of writing, but rather, reflects the lack of coherence and evidence of clear leadership at a national level in this area.

Such is the breadth of the subject area that there are, inevitably, some key areas which cannot be covered in any substantive way within this particular work. For example, the increasingly complex legal environment within which public services seek to manage and also police the application of information and knowledge assets, demands a major textual analysis in its own right. For, just as this preface opened with some reflection upon the implications of the American election debâcle of 2000, so it must draw towards a conclusion with an acknowledgement that the acts of terrorism perpetrated against the USA on 11 September 2001, will have a major impact upon a global public service reform agenda. Information sharing, issues of information security and knowledge exchange have all moved centre stage in response to nations recognising that terrorism does not respect borders and that technology may be harnessed for the most negative of uses.

The intention of this text is therefore to raise questions in the mind of its readership by providing opportunities for detailed analysis of both issues of policy and of operation in applied contexts. Thus key questions should emerge around the challenge of delivering the vision, such as do we understand what this actually is, has it ever been fully articulated and do our public services have the capacity and capabilities to move such an agenda forward?

Consideration of each of the contributions to this work should provide valuable input to the emergence of public services which are reflective of information society and knowledge economy aspirations.

Eileen M. Milner

Acknowledgements

When setting out the aims and objectives of this text, a key priority for myself as the editor was to ensure that a high proportion of the contributions came from those who had been influential in driving forward public service reform and were closely associated with the delivery of change. That this aspiration has been achieved, is a testament to the willingness of the group of thought leaders whose contributions make up this work, to share their ideas and experiences with a wider audience. The somewhat hackneyed adage that the best person to do something important is someone who already has rather too much on their plate, certainly holds true for each of those whose work is shared in this text. I am therefore indebted to each of my colleagues on this project, their commitment and energy for this project has been unfailing. They too would also, I am sure, like to thank all of those who supported them in preparation of their contributions.

A special word of thanks must also go to Edwina Welham and her editorial team at Routledge. The patience and kindness shown, as well as the encouragement provided has made this project an almost entirely positive one to work on.

Thanks also to Eunice Delaney and to John O'Brien whose support made possible the co-operation, at the most senior levels, of the government of the Irish Republic.

Bringing this text to fruition has been a slightly delayed process due to the arrival in the editor's life of a new critic, a daughter, Isabel. As opportunities for public thanks are rare, I would like to take this opportunity to thank Ed Neale, Sheila Skillen, Naomi Gallagher, Helena Hughes and the dedicated team of staff at Bedford Hospital Trust who ensured that everything did turn out well in the end.

Chapter 1

Delivering the vision

An introduction

Eileen M. Milner

Public services: fast, flexible and friendly?

When Kanter argued in the 1990s that successful organisations were characterised by their ability to be 'fast, friendly and flexible', it is likely that her views of best practice had not been substantially informed by observation of such traits in the public services. (Kanter 1990: iii). Public services by their very nature have not been predisposed to speed of delivery, rather they have typically been viewed as being inward facing, overly bureaucratic and focused rather more on procedure than delivery. Flexibility also, is not a noted public service trait, with complex models of governance producing over time, deeply entrenched views of service domains with overtly territorial characteristics predominating. Having a capacity to be welcoming, easy to access and generally inclusive in their approach to all strata within society, are similarly, characteristics that may not be redolent with service users actual experience of engagement with public sector organisations.

However, governments who espouse ambitions to be at the forefront of developments in the creation of an information society and knowledge economy, generally do so with only partial understanding of the way in which a focus upon reengineering public services can provide a powerful catalyst for being at the forefront of such developments. Therefore, the focus of this chapter, is to provide a blueprint for public service developments which is somewhat more grounded in acknowledgement of key inhibitors and barriers, than is often the case when, for example, these profound issues of service reengineering are cloaked in the rhetoric of terms such as electronic government or digital democracy. Examples are drawn from the health service arena in the United Kingdom.

What are we seeking to do?

There is no universally agreed 'recipe' for the way in which public services may need to rethink their rationale however, extracting key areas of activity from globally observed practice would suggest that the following four strands are key:

1   The intention to transform the citizen experience of contact with public services to bring about not only more coherent approaches to accessing services, but to ensure that there is ongoing focus upon usability;

2   To enhance the potential for communication, consultation and engagement both internally and externally;

3   Ensuring that key 'back office' functions operate in open environments, such that, where it is desirable, that information can flow seamlessly and invisibly across service boundaries;

4   Where partner organisations have been tasked with delivering services on behalf of governments, that there are sufficient structures in place to ensure that the operational level knowledge and learning assets which are key to ongoing policy formulation, are not lost from the public service 'loop' entirely.

These points, in themselves, represent major challenges for governments. However, further complexity is added, by the fact that for successful outcomes to be achieved there is a fundamental requirement to treat this reform agenda as a coherent whole, rather than as a menu from which selected points can be extracted. Such an approach represents a critical stage in redefining what is meant by public services. A move away, perhaps, from a perception that public services were something that were essentially one-way, delivery-focused mechanisms. A move away also from a view that public services must be packaged into what were once apparently logical 'parcels' of activity and towards a view that what citizens expect in other aspects of life – namely, ease of use and minimum levels of complexity, are reasonable expectations of publicly provided services. Critically also, perhaps, this reform agenda represents a major challenge to the view that externalising key public services, putting the responsibility for delivery into the hands of those operating at some remove from government, is in its current dominant models of operation, likely to substantially move forward an improvement-focused agenda.

The challenge in this chapter is to consider each of the four identified ingredients in the reform and improvement recipe outlined for public services and to provide some reflection upon where barriers to progress and missed opportunities may occur.

Transforming the citizen experience

When considering pronouncements from politicians on the subject of public service reform, it is possible to establish an overriding theme of transformation as being dominant in their aspirations for moving forward in this arena. However, closer scrutiny of what is actually being advocated and precisely where the locus for transformation would in practice reside, is an area that can appear confusing and contradictory. Thus, for example, in the

United Kingdom, there exist targets for public services to achieve higher levels of migration to information and communications technologies (ICT)-mediated service delivery by 2005 (www.cabinet-office.gov.uk/servicefirst). This, it might be argued is a good example of government providing leadership in a key area and embedding political vision into tightly measured performance criteria. However, for such targets to be meaningful they must, above all else, be relevant and challenging. Where, it can be argued, the United Kingdom's 2005 aspirations fall down, is that they have been moved from the macro level of general vision, down to the micro level of delivery units, with little actual focus upon the role of the user and the transformation of their experience of service interaction. The articulation of targets thus becomes somewhat more mechanistic in focus, allowing the gathering of information to dominate, when a truly transformational agenda might be expected to consider in a more creative manner, how information could be more usefully moved through and across public service operations.

Transformation in this context requires, initially at least, the prioritisation of creativity and innovation in the process of public service design. Critical here is the need to consider patterns of human behaviour, to understand emergent priorities and the ways in which citizens engage with others, particularly those who act as service providers. Considering current public service structures and citizen interactions with them will, almost always, provide an imperfect basis upon which to move forward, for innovation and creativity cannot be reliant upon simply asking service users how things might be improved (Milner 2000: 150). To seek to use views of current structures or delivery mechanisms as ready springboards for achieving change is essentially limiting. However, creativity that is capable of underpinning high levels of service transformation, is far more likely to emerge from researching the changing behaviours exhibited by citizens in relation to other aspects of their daily lives. The public service mission in this context has been articulated by the United Kingdom's Prime Minister, Tony Blair:

> Our challenge is to modernise government and raise the quality and accessibility of all our public services. We acknowledge that people leading busy working lives should not be obliged to queue up during the working day to get to the services they are entitled to. They should be able to access services how and when they want. There are some first rate services . . . like NHS Direct, or NHS Walk-in Centres, which show the way forward. We need to build on these examples.
>
> The first-rate public services of tomorrow will respond quickly to the needs and wishes of its users and produce innovative solutions to the problems that emerge. It will reach out to all groups in the community, old and young, men and women, with or without disabilities, of whatever ethic community. It will value its staff and make best use of them.
>
> (Cabinet Office 2001: 1)

Certainly the agenda set out above is transformational in its language, and realistic in its assessment that such a reform agenda remains, at best, a work in progress. Yet, if we consider the two particular examples of good practice alluded to by the Prime Minister in his statement, those of NHS Direct and NHS Walk-in Centres, and measure them against the first of the four tenets of good practice outlined at the commencement of this chapter, we will find that there remains some scope for constructive criticism. The requirement to focus on achieving coherence of the citizen access experience and a prioritisation of usability of service raises important questions in respect of both exemplars. The rationale for both service developments is described as:

> Making health services more accessible to all is a priority for the Government. There are some exciting new initiatives in the National Health Service (NHS) that are making quality healthcare available to people at times to suit them, reinforcing the message that the patient must come first.
>
> (Cabinet Office 2001: 2)

To consider first the case of walk-in centres, the roll out of which commenced in London in January 2000 and which has continued to gather momentum since then, with the inclusion, under this umbrella, from 2001, of dental services operating under the same 'drop in' principle. Such is the level of resource investment in these services and the similar high level of political expectation that surrounds them, that it is worth careful analysis of how they are described by their architects:

> In a number of towns and cities in England patients are able to walk into NHS centres from early morning until late in the evening and get healthcare advice and treatment for minor injuries, illnesses and ailments from professional, experienced NHS nurses – and all without having to make an appointment.
>
> NHS Walk-in Centres have been introduced by the Government to help people who need easy access to flexible services because of their busy lifestyles or particular circumstances. The 40 existing NHS Walk-in Centres can be found in a variety of convenient places, like alongside Accident and Emergency departments of NHS hospitals and some GP practices. Peterborough and Bristol have the first high-street NHS Walk-in Centres and there's even one at Manchester Airport.
>
> NHS Walk-in Centres are open seven days a week, typically from 7.00 a.m. to 10.00 p.m. during the week and 9.00 a.m. to 10.00 p.m. at weekends. They complement local GP and hospital services, offering fast and convenient access to local NHS advice, information and treatment for minor injuries and illnesses such as cuts sprains and minor infections.
>
> (Cabinet Office 2001: 2)

So what can we extract from this in terms of measuring the extent to which these walk-in centres are likely to enhance the overall coherence of the citizen experience of health care? Perhaps the critical question to raise here, is the extent to which such centres form part of a coherent model of health care delivery, exploiting opportunities for seamless engagement with other elements of the complex organisational model which has long been a characteristic of the United Kingdom's NHS. A first concern to raise is to acknowledge that the parameters for delivering health care through such service points must be limited by the current inability to have portable individual health records. That is to say that in the UK, as is the case in many other major countries, citizen health records are not typically access-ible at all service delivery points. The concept of a working model of electronic patient record is embedded in the 2005 targets discussed at the outset of this chapter, however, even if this aspiration is met in full, it is unlikely that by this date, that centres such as this will have access to a full, detailed electronic health record. The reasons for this relate to the com-plexity of the undertaking in seeking to transfer current paper based records and partial electronic holdings, into a uniform set of data which can be contained within one robust system for a population of some sixty million people.

Thus, one may argue that in the short to medium term at least, that the scope for taking on substantive tranches of work from general practitioners and hospital accident and emergency departments staffed by doctors, is limited. The reasons for such limitations arise from the degree of risk that exists when seeking to deliver health care on the basis of having little or no patient-specific information to hand.

So whilst it may certainly be possible to argue that such centres, staffed by highly qualified nurse practitioners adhering to carefully constructed triage procedures, represent a significant step forward in health provision, there must remain significant concerns around the costs and associated benefits resulting from them. To date it has not been possible to identify any empirical research that supports a view that in areas where such centres exist that there has been a resultant decline in pressure on other frontline healthcare services.

Achieving enhanced coherence and improving effectiveness of service in this context, therefore, would appear to be reliant upon having the ability to work with patients on the basis of properly understood case histories. Without access to such information the predominant operational culture is likely to be one of clinical defensiveness, with referral on to other elements of the service model likely to predominate in all but the most straightforward of cases. There are, additionally, dangers inherent in approaches such as the walk-in centre, whereby patterns of behaviour and presentation of certain injuries may not be accurately fed into the patient's health record. This could actually serve to reduce the ability of health professionals to work in the coherent manner aspired to and lead to some actual decline in the overall pattern of patient care. So whilst developments such as these may ostensibly achieve high scores against usability and coherence criteria, the reality may, at this relatively early stage, be somewhat different. Real service enhancement, achieved through creative use of resources, it seems clear, in a context such as health care provision, is only really likely to be realised when there can be confidence that such services are secure in their underpinning operational frameworks.

Developing this theme still further, significant investment in the NHS Direct call centre model represents a response to wider societal exposure to, and acceptance of, remote access service acquisition and delivery, particularly evident in industries such as insurance and financial services. Moving such an approach out into the health care environment certainly represents an ambitious attempt at creating new behaviours and expectations within the citizen community. Allied to these expectations has been an anticipation that roll out of the call centre service would serve to reduce work pressures on general practitioners and hospital accident and emergency departments. However, to date, as for the walk-in centres, no empirical evidence has been produced to support a view that these anticipated reductions in pressure on frontline services had actually come about. Indeed, within the general practitioner community there exists a prevalent view that investment in an area such as this is wasted, with NHS Direct being referred to by many as no more than a political 'gimmick' (Rumbelow 2001).

The damning term 'gimmick' is critical in making any assessment of critical success factors around transformation of public services, be they in the health services or in revenue collection. The UK government is by no means alone in responding to the changes evident in society where rigid barriers and hierarchies are increasingly being broken down and new service offerings developing. The aspiration to transform the experience of accessing and using public services is entirely proper given even cursory understanding of changing behaviours and expectations within large elements of society.

Yet, if we review the key issues emerging from current developments in the United Kingdom's National Health Service, we see that in one instance, that of the drop-in centres, the potential to undertake significant areas of work is critically limited by the lack of an electronic patient record. In the case of the NHS Direct call centre approach, the opportunities for actually impacting on workloads experienced at the frontline of care are limited by the fact that remote diagnosis, on the basis of computerised triage procedures is, at best, such an inexact science that the likelihood of referral on to other parts of the NHS may actually be increased. In both examples it is possible to argue that the reasons a sense of missed opportunity resonates across any analysis, arises from issues related to both opportunities and weaknesses inherent in the application of information and communications technologies. For the drop-in centres, potential is limited by the absence of sufficient patient information. For NHS Direct there appears to have been rather too much expectation invested in the capacity of ICT-mediated diagnostic procedures, without proper realisation that remote risk assessment is likely to increase frontline referral rates rather than to decrease them.

Of course, when discussing the theme of achieving major public service cultural transformation, it is all too easy, particularly when considering an area as emotive as health care, to be largely negative around current developments. However, to be overly critical is to miss a crucial stage in the transformation process, that of actually raising awareness that new offerings can be made and to establish familiarity with their use. Walk-in centres and NHS Direct are, under their present operating parameters certainly limited in scope. However, the networks that are being created and the expectations and behaviours becoming established in their use, should ensure that they serve as ready platforms for moving forward new models of service delivery as the technology becomes available to support such work. Thus, the NHS Direct framework, both the call centres and the web-based presence, should in time be capable of allowing citizens to book appointments with family doctors, hospital services and other community-based health providers. Although limited in its current scope, it may in the medium term come to be seen and accepted as the gateway to health care in the United Kingdom.

Achieving engagement – a dialogue of the deaf?

Allied to the overarching theme of transformation, is an aspiration on the part of politicians and public service strategists to achieve high levels of engagement from both service users and those involved in the delivery process. This, it may be argued, is set against a prevailing climate of public apathy towards politics and issues of governance in general: a view supported by the fact that in the United Kingdom's general election in 2001, some 40 per cent of those eligible to vote opted not to exercise their democratic right. It is possible in this context to argue that it is not key issues of governance, which provide the major disincentive to participate, but rather dissatisfaction with the political process itself.

In response to perceived citizen dissatisfaction it has been argued that a potential way to re-engage people in the democratic process, is to offer opportunities for greater involvement through the use of referendums on specific issues. Globally there exist very many examples of citizens being asked to provide an opinion, via a vote, lodged usually via telephone or secure web-based site, on matters of local and even national importance. This, it is often argued, serves to make political issues more real to citizens by drilling down into matters of personal concern. However, the adoption of such an approach can have unexpected consequences.

In 2000, Bristol, a major city in the United Kingdom, held a public consultation exercise around the setting of a local taxation rate (council tax). Citizens were asked to identify which of three options they preferred, these being to increase the tax above the 1999 rate, to move to a standstill position, or to actually reduce the tax. Each option was prefaced by a scenario of what the consequences would be. In the case of options two and three, dire predictions were made, particularly around the impact on education services and there appeared confidence in the political community that citizens would register public spirited preferences for increases to be allowed. However, this was not the case, and in fact a large majority of those participating showed a preference for a reduction in the level of taxation (Watt 2001). A clear warning perhaps that if you do wish to engage citizens then you must be prepared to be surprised by their responses.

Similarly, in 2001, the Irish Republic was obliged by its constitution to hold a referendum on ratification of a key European Union policy, that of enlargement, contained within the Treaty of Nice. Conducted on a national scale, this referendum was managed in a traditional manner, that is that voting took place by ballot at designated polling stations. Levels of particip-ation were generally poor, but to the apparent surprise of the government, those participating voted against ratification of the Treaty. The response to this from both Irish politicians and those within the wider European Union framework, which requires that all countries must ratify the proposals for enlargement, is that the question will have to be posed again, until such time as the citizens provide the answers required by the politicians! (McGarry 2001).

Certainly the key theme emerging from the two brief examples outlined above is that whilst it is relatively easy to espouse a political agenda which emphasises consultation and engagement, the reality requires a considerable understanding of the complexities of human motivation and behaviour patterns. To be seen to be seeking to involve citizens in policy development issues is laudable and should serve to enhance the credibility of the political process itself. However, to then discount the views of citizens, or seek to set them within a context which explains why the 'wrong answer' came forward, is to potentially damage the democratic process itself. Critically, at a time when established and emerging technologies are beginning to make it possible for rapid and large scale citizen comment to be gained, to mis-understand the consultation and engagement process, is to invite further disenchantment with the process of governance itself.

Allied to the vision of having wider citizen participation in the policy development process, is a view that all strata of the public service workforce should be engaged in developing an improvement-focused agenda. Such an aspiration is closely linked, both in rhetoric and in application, to the quality management theme of empowerment, which was prevalent in the early 1990s. Indeed, authors such as Kanter, mentioned at the outset of this chapter, and management gurus such as Peters, were passionate advocates of the employee knowledge and experience base as being the best route to organisational improvement (Kanter 1990; Peters 1992). However, whilst these prophets talked of team working and the importance of creating time and space for people to meet, the new rules of engagement reverberate with the importance of having widespread access to an organisational intranet. The time and space that empowerment required, has been replaced by an information repository which should have the capacity for becoming a knowledge resource, where public service employees can not only find out things of relevance to their working environment, but also have the capacity for adding their observations, experiences and suggestions.

The very existence of an intranet both within and across public service organisations has satisfied many that a climate for organisational learning is in place. Yet, if one considers the constraints under which certain intranet sites operate, then the mission to learn and improve must be questioned. For example, consider once more emerging practice in the United Kingdom's National Health Service, where an aspiration to create a national electronic library for health exists, with evidence-based contributions from practitioners making up the majority of information available. However, the mechanisms for achieving entry of information on to this site are formal, with proposed items being required to pass through a lengthy process of review (Salsbury 2001). Whilst such procedures may, of course, result in a robust and perhaps academic representation of emerging practice, it may actually serve to limit the scope for learning through exchange of information, experience and ideas to take place. Overly formal, complex editorial guidelines do not readily serve an aspiration to create a resource which engages the interest and participation of a wide range of employee groups.

For the potential of technology to be realised as an internal communication asset, its approach to content must be structured in such a way that it is accessible and obviously useful to those who engage in its use. Paradoxically also, if investing in intranet technology as a means of achieving new ways of working, it is critical to realise that it is all too easy to create groups of employees who are effectively excluded from interaction with such tools. So, for example, in the health care sector, there remain major issues in the NHS around lack of access for frontline and medical staff to intranet-enabled computers. Similarly, employees working almost entirely away from an office base may have the greatest need to access intranet-held information and be amongst those best placed to feed in their observations, yet limited availability of mobile access to such computer-based services, is a critical limitation in enhancing their effectiveness.

The patterns of practice emerging around the areas of consultation and involvement require careful analysis, particularly in respect of the ways in which developments in these areas may serve to establish new behaviours in both internal and external service users. The examples cited within this chapter reflect ambitious aspirations which are often disappointed at the point of application. The reasons for this are not altogether uniform, but may be said to be generally underpinned by a lack of clear focus upon fundamental issues of human and organisational psychology. Added to this there seems little clear evidence of a coherent practice of evaluation emerging across strands of public service innovation in these areas. Improving perform-ance and associated outcomes on the basis of extracting value from practice and experience would appear to be made a critical area of focus if real progress is to be made on achieving an agenda of wider engagement and input.

Seamless information flows: the ultimate re-engineering challenge?

A dominant theme within this chapter and indeed underpinning the rationale for this text is that the promise of information and communication technologies has, to date, often been illusory. Those who eulogise on the prospects for an information society and a knowledge economy typically do so with little or no understanding of the barriers to progress that technology in itself may present. This position is clearly stated by Lynch:

> The digital economy promised to change the way businesses are run. E-business was meant to enable mobility, information sharing and knowledge empowerment. Technology would introduce new efficiencies and new economies of scale. What a seductive vision! But the very foundation of this new economy is flawed.
>
> What is preventing our entry into the new digital Promised Land is paradoxically the very thing that brought us to its borders: computers. Without humans to tell computers how to process the information they store, computers are worthless. This is particularly true when it comes to processing unstructured information and other kinds of human-friendly information. In the past it was enough to simply automate processes, such as generating a payroll or running invoices, through the use of relational databases and forms-based applications. Data was artificially structured and mainly input into a database and that then stored it in a highly structured row and column format. While the data was useless in its raw state, the database provided a means by which the computer could perform business operations on it.
>
> Today the world is not so simple. It is estimated that 80 per cent of business critical information is locked in the content of unstructured information such as text, spreadsheets, Web pages, e-mails, documents and voice . . .
>
> The bottom line is this – the only way to currently deal with the problem of managing unstructured information . . . is to have people manually intervene. The net effect is that, in the Digital Age, we are forced to create digital sweatshops to preprocess the unstructured information . . .
>
> (Lynch 2001: 5)

Whilst the argument outlined here refers to a business context, the challenges for public services are, if anything, still more complex because of the very scale of the information holdings that are likely to be involved. The relational database applications referred to by Lynch, have proliferated throughout public service environments with little or no checks or balances being put in place to ensure that there is any requirement for a focus upon ultimate connectivity between them. Thus, even within a single public service environment there may exist many stand-alone information repositories, much of the value of which is lost through an inability to allow information to flow across technological boundaries.

The creation of a coherent information and communications technology architecture for public services is a key challenge for any nation aspiring to be seen as a key participant in the development of an information society. However, the scale and scope of such an understanding should not be underestimated. What is perhaps ultimately required is leadership, and allied to this, a political mandate and associated authority to bring largely absent levels of prescription to this area. Seamless information flows cannot be achieved in an environment where technology has been put in place to perform limited tasks, but without any capability for operating in more open environments, adding value through extending its core functionality beyond rigid operational boundaries.

To reflect upon the examples drawn from the United Kingdom's health care service discussed earlier in this chapter, significant limitations have already been identified due to the absence of an effective electronic patient record. To develop this still further, at a time when the government of Tony Blair is emphasising the importance of cross-boundary working between services such as health and the social services provided by tiers of local government, there seems little evident strategy in place to ensure that such co-operative endeavours can achieve their true potential due to an absence of any framework to ensure that information sharing can take place as a matter of routine.

Strassman reflects upon these challenges in a largely positive manner, suggesting that the process of achieving an open operating environment with high levels of connectivity is likely to be an evolutionary process. In support of this view he cites the development of telephone communications:

> Any telephone on earth can communicate with any other telephone, regardless of the enormous variety of institutions and technologies that support these connections. Consider the following characteristics of the existing global telephone networks:
>
> • There are over nineteen thousand local phone exchanges, none of them identical. Some still use over fifty years old technology.
> • There are at least fifty thousand different telephone models, made by

hundreds of manufacturers. They vary in function, color, shape, sound and form.

- There are over thirteen-thousand known calling procedures, such as numbering schemes, ringing sequences, dialing protocols, and identification methods.
- There are telephones in one-hundred and ninety countries. Each country has a different legislative and regulatory approach to administering their telephone system.
- Twenty different time zones are recognized when recording of the time of a phone call.
- There are at least twenty different types of government involved in negotiating how to administer international phone traffic.
- Although there are at least four thousand known languages, somehow operators can handle international traffic.
- The system offers the capacity for any one person to talk to any other person.

(Strassman 1995: 489)

The complexity of the international telephone network outlined by Strassman is certainly analogous in its scale to the challenges represented by the plethora of information and communications technologies currently deployed in public service contexts. However, the current delineating difference is that telephony has evolved underpinning, globally adopted analogue and digital standards, through which voice and facsimile transmissions can pass, effectively nullifying, from the perspective of the end user, any differences in operating systems.

Strassman develops his arguments around how a climate of public service connectivity might be achieved through scrutiny of practice in the United States defence services. Stripping his analysis of defence-specific characteristics, it is possible to extract a set of factors which might be generalisable across the whole of public service practice, priorities emerging would be:

- Put in place a single whole of government focus for technical control and configuration management.
- Establish a single systems house for centralised acquisition of hardware and software, the priority here should be upon maximisation of information 'utility', rather than upon the merits of individual applications.
- Provide appropriate guidance on training and development of employees interacting with technologies, the emphasis should be upon ensuring that all appropriate technological capabilities are understood and ultimately utilised.
- Assure interoperability, common operating standards and approaches to security through the creation of a centralised body to monitor levels of integration, testing applications in specific contexts and providing a

locus for exploring levels of usability amongst a variety of user communities. Such a body should also serve as a locus for gathering examples of good practice and promulgating them as appropriate.

- Ensure that there are appropriate back-up procedures in place to minimise any problems arising from system failure.

The challenges articulated here are immense. Fundamentally they challenge a predominant global public service culture where information and communication technologies have been permitted to proliferate without adequate regulation or supervision. Yet, the operational information silos that have evolved as a result of this largely *laissez-faire* approach provide perhaps the biggest barrier to public service reform, which exists today. A typical response from politicians and senior managers to the barriers encountered due to an inability for information to flow seamlessly, is to blame vendor companies for exploiting their position by ensuring non-compatibility with other operating platforms and tools. However, such an attitude is, at best disingenuous, for after all vendors are not responsible for developing the specifications which ultimately lead to the awarding of contracts. Rather, responsibility must lie with those charged with enacting change and purchasing products to help move such an agenda forward. It is for public service managers to articulate exactly what their requirements are and to demonstrate that they have a clear understanding of the requirement to focus on the need for wider engagement with other branches of public service. This, quite simply, has been largely absent from the public service environment and without it, aspirations to be at the forefront of driving forward information society and knowledge economy inspired change agenda, are embedded far more in the rhetoric than in any attainable reality.

Losing our organisational memory

Increasingly, organisations are focusing upon how they might successfully seek to harness the knowledge assets associated with their employees. Typically this may involve requesting or requiring staff to contribute to intranet sites arranged around particular client interactions or project roll-outs, although there are many other models of practice operating in all sectors of the economy. Such activity represents a major acknowledgement of the pivotal role that employees at all levels of an organisation may play in informing the learning and development processes that provide the essential dynamism underpinning successful twenty-first century organisations. However, almost paradoxically, for public services the operating environment is shifting, to such an extent that the structures and cultures emerging may actually militate against any opportunities for such learning and development to be fed into policy and strategy development processes. The potential danger of moving to a model of public service where government is at some remove from the operational aspects, due to outsourcing or partnership arrangements, should not be underestimated.

Governments who advocate the adoption of a position where they are an enabler rather than necessarily a direct provider of public services have typically not acknowledged the fact that they may be absenting themselves from an environment which is most likely to inform their service planning. Even much vaunted partnership agreements typically do not require that knowledge or intelligence accruing through the service delivery process, should automatically be fed into the policy development arm of the body managing the contract on behalf of the public service. Rather, the emphasis to date has been upon ensuring that performance criteria have been put in place, against which often crude measures of baseline performance can be assessed. In terms of accepted modes of contract management this is, of course, standard practice but whether it is wholly appropriate practice in the public service domain is questionable.

However, to identify instances of missed opportunities, as arising in only those organisations that have been subject to some form of externalisation process, is to miss a crucial point. In the commercial sector the management of knowledge has achieved a high profile, largely because it is seen as being a key factor in ensuring that a climate of innovation and improvement is created and sustained. In the public services there has been traditionally far less recognition of the importance of constantly seeking to learn and to extract value from analysis of learning opportunities. The challenge, and perhaps the critical paradox now, is that in a climate when public services are being called upon to innovate and to develop new modes of user-centred working, they are increasingly seeing their key employee assets being transferred to agencies or organisations at some remove from their direct control.

The concept of organisational memory is an important one in any context where there is an improvement-focused change agenda in place. The reference to *memory* relates primarily to the value of experience and expertise that has been developed over time, where knowledge has accrued that can provide valuable indicators of how an organisation may learn from past practice in particular. A key concern in emergent modes of public service delivery and associated cultures is that such assets are lost, ignored, or rendered less than effective through employee disenchantment. Crude analysis of the global public service environment reveals a disquieting reliance upon external consultants to provide crucial service re-engineering input. Typically there is little or no emphasis placed upon engaging those who have been involved in the service delivery process in developing new ways of working. Such an approach is, in itself perverse when set alongside the attitudes and value set suggested by information society and knowledge economy aspirations, where real value is seen to reside in people.

Achieving greater utilisation of organisational memory, extraction and exploitation of knowledge assets, or put more crudely maximising the value of the employee base of public services, represents both a challenge and an opportunity. Here there can be no reliance upon immediate technology delivered solutions but rather, there is a requirement for a fundamental reappraisal of how public services learn and develop.

Fast, flexible and friendly . . . delivering the vision

The change agenda set out in this chapter is an ambitious one, requiring far greater emphasis than has typically been the case to date, upon achieving coherence across the range of public service offerings. The requirement for coherence and connectivity is paramount and it must be evident at the very highest levels of idea and policy generation. Public services that operate within commonly understood models of what an information society and knowledge economy should be, will have to be different. A position where multiple and fractured service entry points is the norm, is simply no longer sustainable as citizens' expectations begin to be set by their engagement with other areas of service provision not in the public service domain. The examples contained within this chapter demonstrate that there is certainly a sense of challenge and opportunity underpinning major swathes of public service reform currently ongoing. However, careful analysis of the operational limitations associated with such developments reveals that there is something close to a vacuum of understanding around key limitations, which exist, in these emergent structures.

An overarching theme of this text lies in its focus upon delivery of quantifiable change rather than relying upon the purely aspirational strands of public service reform. At the outset of this chapter Kanter's exhortation that organisations should seek to be 'fast, flexible and friendly' was explored within a context which identified that such traits were not normally associated with public services (Kanter 1990: iii). It is appropriate to question at the conclusion of this chapter whether the service innovations referred to, indicate that there is fundamental and far-reaching change being enacted within the public service environment. However, the answer to such a question would, essentially, have to be multi-faceted if it were to have any wider credibility. Public services as described in this chapter are certainly seeking to innovate, they are clearly working in new ways and offering citizens routes to services which may be more convenient, more attuned to lifestyles and less intimidating than in the past. Such achievements must not be underestimated for they may represent the building blocks of new public service cultures and ethos which once established in the minds of the citizen will build demand and momentum for wider change.

However, a multi-faceted response to the question set is required and whilst acknowledging the considerable achievements already attained, it is also important to realise that there are critical limitations contained within the approaches adopted so far. The four-point change agenda set out within this chapter is a challenging and ambitious one, requiring as it does fundamental realignment of the way in which information, knowledge, technology and people are utilised within the public services framework. In none of the examples discussed is there clear evidence that each of these issues has been addressed with the rigour required, nor is there any clear indication that, as yet, there is any sense of connectivity between each of these key elements. The model of reform which seems to dominate in the examples cited here, appears to be disconnected in too many ways from any over-arching strategy focused upon bringing about a platform for coherent and ongoing change and innovation. Fast, flexible and friendly public services may be emerging as pockets of practice, yet the challenge of actually delivering wide-ranging reform remains, in analysis of practice in the United Kingdom at least, an issue requiring both understanding and leadership at the very highest levels.

References

Cabinet Office (2001) *Open All Hours – A Report on Extended Service Hours,* London: Cabinet Office Modernising Public Services.

Kanter, R.M. (1990) *When Giants Learn to Dance,* New York: Touchstone.

Lynch, M. (2001) *Automating the Digital Economy, Autonomy Annual Report and Accounts 2000*, Cambridge: Autonomy Corp.

McGarry, P. (2001) 'Which question shall we answer?' Dublin: *The Irish Times*, Online. Available HTTP: http://www.ireland.com (15 June 2001).

Milner, E. (2000) *Managing Information and Knowledge in the Public Sector,* London: Routledge.

Peters, T. (1992) *Liberation Management: Necessary Disorganization for the Nanosecond Nineties,* London: Macmillan.

Rumbelow, H. (2001) 'Research calls into question the benefits of NHS Direct', London: *The Times*, Online. Available HTTP: http://www.TheTimes.com (4 July 2001).

Salsbury, K. (2001) 'Developing frameworks for managing knowledge in the National Health Service', unpublished Phd working paper, University of North London.

Strassman, P. (1995) *The Politics of Information Management: Policy Guidelines,* Connecticut: Information Economics Press.

Watt, N. (2001) 'Hague promises council tax referendums', London: *The Guardian*, Online. Available HTTP: http://www.SocietyGuardian.co.uk (20 May 2001).

Chapter 2

Seven e-government milestones

Janet Caldow

As electronic government comes of age around the world, leadership remains at the core of success, beginning with the definition of e-government itself. Leaders who define e-government in a narrow sense – simply moving services online – miss larger opportunities which will determine competitive advantage in the long run. Indeed, by the end of the decade, what will constitute competitive advantage? Certainly not renewing a licence online. By then, online government services will be as commonplace as ATM machines are today. Online services will no longer be noteworthy, distinguishing one government from another, but will have become part of a baseline expectation of service delivery. Given such a scenario, governments today have no choice but to aggressively pursue an all-encompassing shift from traditional to online service delivery. To do nothing places them in jeopardy of falling below minimally acceptable standards of service.

Therefore, if online service delivery is only the ante to get into e-government, what then will set governments apart, elevating e-government as a competitive advantage? What are leaders to do? A broader grasp of e-government is imperative for leaders to position their governments, citizens, businesses and communities for sustainable strategic advantage.

Seven leadership milestones are integral to both becoming an e-government and running an e-government. Achieving these milestones, it may be argued, creates competitive advantage in both instances:

Milestone one:	integration
Milestone two:	economic development
Milestone three:	e-democracy
Milestone four:	e-communities
Milestone five:	intergovernmental
Milestone six:	policy environment
Milestone seven:	next generation internet

These milestones are neither discrete nor sequential in nature. Each milestone has equal priority, contributing to the cumulative attainment of the others. Concurrent activity among the seven areas are required from the beginning. So, how do you attain e-government? Imagine a team of seven horses pulling a wagon. Each horse is connected to each other, as well as to the wagon. Unless all seven horses are pulling, the wagon cannot pass the milestones necessary to reach its destination. For example, to achieve milestone seven, broadband application pilots should be set into motion now in order to be ready for 'prime time' when high-speed access reaches critical mass. Collectively, these milestones require a common underlying management foundation and investment in strategy, collaboration, governance structures, financial investment, human resources, and partnerships. Without this leadership foundation, progress will be limited in overall impact and at best, will be fragmented.

Milestone one: integration

Process integration and technology integration mark the achievement of milestone one. Most governments have already recognised the fact that effective citizen services are delivered independently of existing organisational structures. Some call it one-stop shopping, one window, or refer to a central entry point as a portal. This approach is designed to allow citizens to access services without having to know which department handles the service. Put simply, instead of a list of departments to click, citizens find a list of services to click. This is undoubtedly welcome progress. However, behind the citizen interface, most of today's portals actually transfer the transaction to the individual agency and its technology systems for processing. The bottom line is that each service still has a one-to-one relationship with the department that offers it – reserve a tennis court, renew a realtor's licence, pay a fine, file taxes. Thus, such services are not quite as progressive as they might first appear. This is not real process integration of government operations. Indeed, what happens if the process involves several agencies? Governments can learn from 'dotcom' start-ups that launched elaborate websites to sell direct to customers, compared with companies that have transformed their existing offerings into e-businesses. Just as clicking on something to buy is different from using the internet to run a business so clicking on a licence renewal is different from using the internet to run a government.

It is likely that most people have been victims of poorly integrated processes and services in both public and private sectors. Personally, I have four policies with the same insurance company, one of the largest in this sector in the United States. Yet, the company mails to me as a customer four different bills, at four different times, with four different payment configurations. Worse still, each bill is only identified with a policy number. You could argue that in terms of managing the customer relationship more effectively, such organisations would acknowledge that customers generally have better things to do than to memorise four 16-digit policy numbers.

Reflecting on how public services might learn from such practice, the Texas Comptroller of Public Accounts office established the e-Texas Commission to find ways to reduce the number of touch points required to establish a business in Texas. They identified that to open a dry cleaning shop in Texas requires interaction with five state agencies – the Department of Licensing and Regulation, the Texas Natural Resource Conservation Commission, the Comptroller of Public Accounts, the Texas Workforce Commission and the Texas Department of Transportation. Authorisation from each department is required in order to establish and transact business in Texas. In addition, the dry cleaner must comply with regulations at the Federal level – the Environmental Protection Agency, the Department of Labor and the Department of Transportation. Taking a slightly different sector, a food retailer is subject to nine state regulatory agencies, seventeen different types of state licences, and various statewide inspection processes.

Why is it so difficult to conduct simple business? It can be argued that such complexity occurs because cross-boundary operations, organisational structures, and information technology systems are not integrated. So, returning to my own experience of insurance services, it is obvious that the car insurance division only cares about cars and that the house insurance division is only interested in houses. The company has a website where you can click on either car or house insurance. However, from the policy owner's perspective, there is no apparent attempt at integration for total insurance needs. Each division operates in isolation. Each division has different technology platforms with databases and applications that are incompatible with other divisions. Perhaps most astonishing of all, the company as a whole probably does not have the technology infrastructure to handle integration.

Integration is core to running either a business or a government in today's digital environment. E-business is a business model focusing on business relationships at the enterprise level powered by electronic interfaces among internal divisions, business partners, employees and customers. The combination of interfaces among individual legacy systems, enterprise level applications, and breakthrough internet-based technologies for external customer and supplier use make e-business achievable, affordable and mandatory for competitiveness. To achieve milestone one, governments need to learn to use the internet to run public services.

In reality does this mean that there is a need to look 'backwards' by moving discrete services online on a common portal? The answer to this is probably yes. Portals, despite certain key limitations, do generally represent visible quick wins, garnering citizen support, cutting transaction time and costs, and improving levels of convenience to the user. Governments in this context must be aggressive, committing to moving the bulk of services online within a challenging time-frame. However, they should not stop there. Responsible and far-sighted administrations should demand that each functional area develop the discipline to look at interactions from a 'total customer experience' perspective. Such a customer-focused audit exercise should point to the need to create a public service framework that is a truly 'networked organisation' with a high priority being placed upon attaining logical work flow linkages across departments and information technology systems.

The state of Manitoba in Canada discovered the benefits of focusing upon such linkages. Efforts are now underway to eliminate duplication of services and to bridge gaps between logical groupings of operations using technology as the intermediary. Their Better Systems Initiative calls for a consolidated view for the citizens it serves, accessible from a broad range of electronic communications devices such as telephones, PCs, interactive TV and electronic kiosks. Integration is the key. Family Services, in partnership with IBM Canada Ltd, performed the necessary process re-engineering, system development, and infrastructure to integrate both provincial services and City of Winnipeg services into one common management system. Another technology platform now integrates taxation, licencing, royalties and miscellaneous revenue services, permitting a common system of revenue collection and receipt across a number of functional departments.

For the same reasons, the province of Ontario established a unique chief information officer structure to facilitate cross-boundary integration. The chief information officer for the province manages infrastructure, standards and strategy. Seven other chief information officers serve clusters of related ministries. These innovations were pivotal in helping to break down traditional departmental boundaries.

Integration requires both process integration and technical integration. The customer experience drives both. A business perceives the task 'open a business' as a single objective with government, whereas government perceives it as multiple steps with multiple transactions. A customer perceives 'pay my insurance bill' as a single transaction, whereas the insurance company perceives it as 'bill each policy type'. These are process integration issues which demand management intervention.

Underneath process integration is technical infrastructure integration. What exactly does this mean? Certainly, leaders need to understand the infrastructure integration side of the equation, at least from a high level, in order to provide direction. However, key back-office operations, such as a data centre, are likely professionally staffed, follow disciplined operating procedures around security, availability, reliability, scaleability and performance standards. Yet, web servers throughout your organisation probably do not have such established structures with which to work. It is possible to argue that today's infrastructure is simply not up to the task of the tremendous growth in use that is anticipated, for example in the medium term it is estimated that there will be, ten times the number of people connected to the internet; 100 times the current network speed; 1000 times the number of connected devices; and a million times the data. Calculate those numbers across any public service structure – can the technical infrastructure handle it? Not only do your databases and applications need to talk to each other, now the engines that drive them – the PCs, web servers, LANs, networks also have to attain a new level of standards.

Today, most e-businesses are planning 99.9999 per cent availability. That means systems are guaranteed to be up and handle the load 99.9999 per cent of the time. When e-government comes of age, you cannot afford to have 90 per cent availability, that represents the equivalent of closing all your government offices a half day per week during normal business hours. What's more, in the e-government world, the working week is no longer 40 hours, it is 168 hours: 24 hours a day, 7 days a week. Surveys indicate that most e-government services are accessed between the hours of 8.00 p.m. and 2.00 a.m. Whilst a data centre may be open and staffed all night, the web masters from the recreation or licencing department are probably home in bed asleep! E-government represents a complete change in established mindsets about how you run things.

In the context of integration it is also worth considering what might be referred to as 'loads and bottlenecks'. Within the next 5 years, bandwidth will increase 150 times. When such high speed access is commonplace the internet will not be to blame for slow response or crashes because of seasonal peaks, uneven traffic and increasing demand. All the stress will be transferred to servers and networks. Consider also the portal and all the service transactions pushed out to separate web sites, and the technical challenges become clear. Fundamentally, the more agencies and servers involved, the less reliability there will be if they are not part of a disciplined management structure. If just one server goes down in any one of the agencies at any step along the process, you could not complete, for example, a business permit application. Thus, each web server needs to be integrated into the same standard IT operating procedures prioritising security, availability, reliability and performance.

Another level of integration involves enterprise systems, such as finance, human resources, tax/revenue and payroll. Countless organisations migrated to enterprise resource planning systems (ERP), or purchased package systems, to be Y2K compliant instead of rewriting 20-year-old applications. Customer relationship management (CRM) has also become increasingly important in this arena. CRM serves constituents through the phone, in person, via a PC, over the internet, using a personal digital assistant (PDA), or by mail with a single view to the customer. Database management has evolved to data warehousing (for data sharing) and to data mining. Most data mining initiatives (searching and comparing data from various sources) in government are for fraud and abuse prevention purposes. An example is cross-checking tax bills and payments from various departments to see if taxes are refunded from one system, while outstanding balances are due in another. In such contexts it is possible to argue that E-commerce applications (online renewal and payment for licences, for example) came of age, extending legacy platforms and functionality without necessarily changing the legacy systems themselves. Now we have new technical silos and these too need to be integrated. For example, e-commerce web sites should be part of overall customer relationship management. Currently it is likely that such services are handled separately. Data mining capability should extend across ERP systems and e-commerce sites, so you have a grasp of how your enterprise is actually functioning as a whole. This capability is known as business intelligence or knowledge management. Integration when framed in such a way, has the potential to provide a whole new management resource across government.

Significant investment is required to achieve viable levels of integration. Hardware, software, security, scaleability, reliability, skilled personnel, integration of process and technical infrastructure – all are fundamental in running an e-government. There is also a requirement to acknowledge that achievement of such goals cannot come from reliance upon today's environment built for a physical government. Decades and even in some cases centuries were spent in establishing processes and procedures to operate physical governments. Now, however, we are shifting to a brand new paradigm. The good news is that the savings, rewards and returns far outstrip the investment required.

Milestone two: economic development

On the road to e-government, Digital Age economic development generally has five dimensions – leveraging small- and medium-sized businesses; education; attracting high-tech industry; access to technology infrastructure and having a business-friendly government.

Economic development once focused on attracting a few large corporations to build plants and bring jobs to a nation or region Although still a building block, the tide has turned toward small- and medium-sized businesses – the fastest growing economic sector worldwide. Governments may have from hundreds to potentially tens of thousands of small businesses within their boundaries. If each one has the opportunity to grow into a 'clicks and mortar' enterprise, and adds just one new job per year, the result is likely to be overall healthy economic growth.

What do these small businesses need and how can government leaders help? To transform into e-business, small- and medium-sized companies need affordable expertise and technology – web development, e-commerce applications, hosting, and high-speed internet access. Individually, small companies have little bargaining power. However, together, through organised aggregation of demand, negotiated affordable packages for these capabilities can become a reality – perhaps a citywide or statewide services contract for small businesses. Governments, in collaboration or working through private and nonprofit sectors can facilitate such bargaining power.

Whilst helping small- and medium-sized companies become e-businesses is one thing, actually establishing brand recognition is quite another. In the economic shift to e-business, small and medium businesses are losing customers to big, heavily advertised internet brands. Search engines, in the main, are still primitive and frustrating. In this climate the likelihood is that a local resident will go directly to a known internet brand instead of searching for local e-businesses. When an out-of-state online transaction occurs, lost sales taxes are only one part of the problem. Those companies are also not paying state income taxes or business licence fees. Further, they do not employ your resident citizens, their employees are not shopping at your local shopping centres. The potential for economic growth (or loss thereof) associated with an online purchase should not be underestimated. The solution is not simply changing sales tax laws if these are applicable but rather more about helping businesses to get online and then facilitating their operation by helping them to get connected with your citizens. One way to do this is building upon milestone one – integrate from your citizens' perspectives. Provide easy citizen access from the government portal to reach local businesses. Feature a 'small e-business of the week' on the website. Have a robust enough portal, and these small businesses will enjoy not only brand awareness amongst residents, but will enjoy access to new customers and business partners outside the local area. This effectively bridges 'local' to 'global' for business development and economic growth.

Building a competitive workforce to fill newly created jobs is the companion strategy to leveraging small businesses and attracting industry. The Information Technology Association of America estimates, in the United States alone, ten million jobs are associated with the internet; and that within this market that 850,000 vacancies exist. People no longer have to work where they live. A digital workforce is emerging where jobs can be filled anywhere in the world. This dramatic and growing shortage of skills affects every country, every state, every city. Jobs displaced in the digital economy are being replaced with new internet-related jobs at much higher salaries. Education, of course, is key here and is why it has become a number one priority of government leaders everywhere. An education system that produces a competitive workforce is undeniably core to economic growth. For example, governments are rethinking degree programme caps to encourage more science, mathematics, engineering and technology graduates.

Governments also need strategies to attract new knowledge workers and high-tech businesses into their areas. The Commonwealth of Virginia has been particularly successful in attracting and growing a high-tech industry base. Today, nearly 50 per cent of the world's internet traffic flows through northern Virginia. The area is home to America Online and thousands of other high-tech companies. Fortune magazine referred to Virginia's 'netplex' as a dense pattern of interaction and partnering among firms in a highly dynamic telecommunications industry, a rapidly emerging internet industry and what is probably the most highly developed concentration of systems engineering capabilities in the world.

Leadership for Virginia's strategy has spanned nearly two decades and several governors' administrations. In 1984, the Center for Innovative Technology was established as a nonprofit organisation designed to enhance the research and development capability of the state's major research universities. Ten years later, the CIT adopted a new mission that measured success in terms of jobs created, companies created and competitiveness created for Virginia's businesses. Within 3 years of the new focus, Virginia businesses created 9,854 new jobs, 222 new companies and $278 million in competitiveness gains. In 1998 another 10,609 jobs were created, 132 new companies and $1.9 billion in competitiveness. Virginia has become a 'hot spot' of technology because of its relentless focus on developing the workforce, creating the infrastructure, maintaining an entrepreneurial climate and deploying technology. Governor Gilmore, elected in 1997, has made technology a top issue of his administration. In his first year in office, he created the Commission on Information Technology, charged with developing a comprehensive technology policy for the Commonwealth. The governor issued an executive order creating the nation's first Secretary of Technology. In 1998, Donald Upson was appointed to that post, responsible for coordinating public sector information technology resources, whilst also working with Virginia's fast growing information technology private sector. In 1999, the state's internet Policy Act was signed into law, becoming a model for other states.

As a result of these leadership strategies, venture capital attracted into the area grew from $400 million in 1997 to $1.6 billion in 1999. Between 1992 and 1998, the number of technology firms increased an average of 10.2 per cent annually. A 2000 report entitled *Technology in Virginia's Regions* (Commonwealth of Virginia 2000) reported 4,324 technology firms in Virginia employing 386,241 people. *Virginia Economic Trends* (Commonwealth of Virginia 1999) reported in first quarter, 1999, the average earnings per technology employee was $65,021, or almost twice the state's overall average. Two new task forces, created in 2000 by the Governor and Secretary of Technology, take the strategy even further. 'From Main Street to E-Street' and the 'E-Communities' task forces are exploring ways to engage every town, city, county, business and citizen in the Commonwealth, both rural and urban, to reap the benefits of economic growth in a global digital economy. By 2003, Virginia is expected to have nearly 423,000 technology workers, earning $26.4 billion. Effective leadership in these areas is clearly bringing immense benefits to Virginia.

Creating a business friendly climate extends to traditional government-to-business interaction. How easy is it to research traditional economic development information – available office space, transportation systems, air quality, crime rates, workforce statistics, school systems, residential housing costs? Is it in one convenient place?

Businesses typically have many more interactions with their governments each year than the average citizen. Therefore, another new decision criterion for deciding where to locate a business is whether a government demonstrates it can move at the speed of business. E-businesses operate in compressed time. If it takes 120 days for a government to approve a building permit when the business has to be operational within one web year (90 days), logic dictates the business will decide to locate in another jurisdiction that is more business friendly.

Milestone three: e-democracy

The manifestation of e-democracy stretches across the spectrum of democratic process. No e-government vision is complete without some attention being paid to issues of digital democracy. The spectrum ranges from voter registration, voting, public opinion polling, communication among elected representatives and their constituencies, universal access to technology, wired legislative bodies and legislative processes that encourage greater citizen participation. Online hearings, submitting expert testimony online, opinion polling and open communication and information provide opportunities for real-time participation throughout the democratic process – not simply disseminating information after the fact, which represents the greatest cultural change of all.

From John Locke to Thomas Jefferson, the foundation of democracy is an informed and engaged citizenry. Increasingly governments receive 'high marks' for making information accessible online, yet much more needs to be done. Improved two-way communication between constituents and representatives and better ways for citizens to engage in the legislative process are all part of becoming an e-government. Clift's 'Top Ten E-Democracy To Do List' offers good advice on how to integrate digital democracy into e-government strategies:

1   Announce all public meetings online in a systematic and reliable way. Include the time, place, agenda and information on citizen testimony, participation, or observation options. Use the internet to build trust in in-person democracy.
2   Put a 'Democracy Button' on your site's top page which brings them to a special section detailing the agencies/government units purpose and mission, top decision-makers, links to enabling laws, budget details and other accountability information. Share real information that help a citizen better understand the legitimacy of your government agency and powers, and how to best influence the policy course of the agency. This could include links to the appropriate parliamentary or local council committees and bodies.
3   Implement 'Service Democracy'. Yes, most citizens simply want better, more efficient access to service transactions and information products

your agency produces. Learn from these relationships. Actively use comment forms, online surveys, citizen focus groups to garner the input required to be a responsive e-government. Don't automate services that people no longer want or need. Use the internet to learn about what you can do better and not just as a one-way self-service tool designed to limit public interaction and input.

4 End the 'Representative Democracy Online Deficit'. With the vast majority of government information technology spending focused on the administrative side of government, the representative institutions from the local level on up to the federal government are growing increasingly weak. Invest in the technology and communications infrastructure of those institutions designed to represent the people.

5 Internet-enable existing representative and advisory processes. Create 'virtual committee rooms' and public hearings that allow in-person events to be available in totality via the internet. Require in-person handouts and testimony to be submitted in HTML for immediate online availability to those watching or listening on the internet or via broadcasting. Get ready to datacast such items via digital television. Encourage citizens to also testify via the internet over video conferencing and allow online submission of written testimony. The most sustainable 'e-democracy' activities will be those incorporated into existing and legitimate governance processes.

6 Embrace the two-way nature of the internet. Create the tools required to respond to e-mail in an effective and timely manner. E-mail is the most personal and cherished internet tool used by the average citizen. How a government deals with incoming e-mail and enables access to automatic informational notices based on citizen preferences will differentiate popular governments from those that are viewed as out of touch. Have a clear e-mail response policy and start by auto-responding with the time and date received, the estimated time for a response, what to do if none is received, and a copy of their original message. Give people the tools to help hold you accountable.

7 Hold government-sponsored online consultations. Complement in-person consultations with time-based, asynchronous online events (1 to 3 weeks) that allow people to become educated on public policy issues and interact with agency staff, decision-makers, and each other. Online consultations must be highly structured events designed to have a real impact on the policy process. Don't do this for show. The biggest plus with these kinds of events is that people may participate in their own time from homes, schools, libraries and workplaces and greater diversity of opinions, perspectives and geography can increase the richness of the policy process. Make clear the government staff response permissions to allow quick responses to informational queries. Have a set process to deal with more controversial topics in a very timely (24-48 hours)

fashion with direct responses from decision-makers and top agency staff. Do this right and your agency will want to do this at least quarterly every year, do it wrong the first time and it will take quarter of a century to build the internal support for another try. Check on the work in Canada, the Netherlands, Sweden and United Kingdom in particular and you'll discover governments are up to some exciting work.

8   Develop e-democracy legislation. Tweak laws and seek the budgetary investments required to support governance in information age. Not everything can be left voluntary – some government entities need a push. What is so important that government must be required to comply? There is a limit to what can be squeezed out of existing budgets. Even with the infrastructure in place the investment in the online writers, communicators, designers, programmers and facilitators must be increased to make internet-enhanced democracy something of real value to most citizens and governments alike.

9   Educate elected officials on the use of the internet in their representative work. Get them set up technologically and encourage national and international peer-to-peer policy exchanges among representatives and staff. Be careful to prevent use of this technology infrastructure for incumbency protection. Have well-designed laws or rules to prevent use of technology and information assets in unknown ways. Don't be overly restrictive, but e-mail gathered by an elected official's office shouldn't suddenly be added to a campaign e-mail list.

10 Create open source democracy online applications. Don't waste tax dollars on unique tools required for common governmental IT and democracy needs. Share your best in-house technology with other governments around the world. Leverage your service infrastructure, be it proprietary or open source, for democratic purposes. With vast resources being spent on making administrative government more efficient, a bit of these resources should be used 'inefficiently.' Democracy is the inefficiency in decision-making and the exercise of power required for the best public choices and outcomes.

(Clift 2000)

Legislative bodies are beginning to understand how technology can transform themselves as members gather to debate and vote in floor sessions. In most cases, the predominant use of any technology inside legislative bodies is limited to electronic systems to tabulate floor votes. Even then, output from these ageing systems must be manually entered many times into other systems for reporting purposes and then translated into a different format for posting to websites. New technologies allow legislators – during formal sessions – to communicate silently with staff back in their offices, conduct real-time research on issues on the internet, negotiate terms with members of their own or opposing parties, while debate continues. Wisconsin and other governments have begun to outfit all legislators with laptop computers.

Components of the electoral process – campaigning, communication with constituents and the media, coordination of volunteers, solicitation and collection of campaign contributions, voter registration and voting – are also facets of the e-democracy milestone. According to a September, 2000, Council for Excellence in Government report, '*E-Government: The Next American Revolution*', nearly 59 per cent of Americans oppose voting online (Hart 2000). However, given the experiences during the November 2000, United States' presidential election, clearly voting reform is an issue.

In the United States, over 3,000 counties currently deploy voting at over 200,000 polling sites. Technologies utilised range from punchcard, optical scanning, lever, direct recording electronics to paper ballots. Many of these are ageing or obsolete systems. Few, if any, standards exist, even within individual states. Security, privacy and sheer infrastructure issues will delay widespread 'i-voting', or voting over the internet. Rather voting systems are likely to evolve first through 'e-voting' solutions, or more reliable electronic voting systems located at the polling place. However, upgrading voting systems requires a leadership commitment to funding and standards.

The collection and counting of votes is only one part of the challenge. Many times, changes made to traditional voter registration systems (such as address changes) are not processed in time for election day. Redundant voter data may exist in several locations within a state (if a voter moves). These are straightforward database design and integration issues, which are relatively easy and inexpensive to correct. Many jurisdictions also overlook the importance of human interface design. This step is critical whether the interface is between a voter and a paper ballot, a machine, or a computer screen.

Milestone four: e-communities

Government is intrinsic to community life and well-being in fundamental ways. Public safety, public health, parks and recreation, elderly and youth services being tangible examples. Yet, government is also integral to the very basic quality of life, including issues such as equal opportunity, education, diversity and even seasonal celebrations. Any commitment to e-government should, therefore, extend its remit to include some focus upon enriching the communities government serves. Put simply, people are not just citizens of a government, they are parents, families, volunteers, neighbours, consumers, students, sports enthusiasts, senior citizens, children and members of religious and social institutions – forming communities of interest within a geo-graphic community. Together they weave the rich tapestry of an often diverse geo-community, the cornerstone of society. In this context, it is important to recognise that the definition of community at the local government level is different from a state, provincial or national community, but each has important sociological implications. Across all strata of government, facilitating and supporting e-communities should be a key area of strategic focus for those involved in delivering e-government.

Internet technologies offer unparalleled opportunities for government to enhance communities. Once the e-government technology infrastructure is in place to offer online services through a website portal, the marginal cost of adding additional components becomes very small.

In February 1999, the Government of Canada announced a nationwide Smart Communities initiative (Government of Canada 2000). Sixty million dollars over 3 years are earmarked for one Smart Community demonstration project in each province, one in the north, and one in an Aboriginal community. These projects are designed to explore and test ways in which information and communication technologies can be harnessed by communities across Canada to support economic development and to enrich community life for Canadians. Within the confines of this work, Canada defines a smart community as follows:

> A Smart Community is a community with a vision of the future that involves the use of information and communication technologies in new and innovative ways to empower its residents, institutions and regions as a whole.

Communities around the world are responding to the needs of their citizens by discovering new ways of using information and communication technologies for economic, social and cultural development. Communities and countries that take advantage of these new technologies will create jobs and economic growth as well as improve the overall quality of life within their communities.

Since 1992, Naestved in Denmark has launched an impressive series of integrated e-community initiatives spanning government, private and commercial interests with the intention of attracting investment, bringing the information society one step closer to reality, and plugging into the heart of the emerging digital economy. Beginning in 1992, with a new mayor and a new vision, an e-community groundwork was laid with an intranet. A Lotus Notes platform (collaboration software) for employees citywide was installed in 1994. In 1995, CityNet was created, a joint venture between Naestved, Cable TV and TeleDenmark, which provided cheap, high-speed internet access to any household or business within city limits. In 1996, NaestvedNet (a semiprivate company owned by the regional newspaper, telecompany and municipality) drove the creation of the NaestvedNet Business Council to stimulate growth of local businesses. The business council offered education, technical support, and affordable web services for small and medium businesses wishing to get online. In 1997, the city website (www.naeskom.dk)

was designed to provide self-services. 'New Pathway' centres were also estab-lished to serve the physically impaired, senior citizens and the unemployed. PCs were installed in all libraries and youth data centres opened. In 1999, Naestved was approved as an EU pilot of Open Digital Administration, to implement digital signatures using Tivoli public key infrastructure giving citizens secure access to case processing applications, including intelligent forms (data automatically filled in). In 2000, Naestved created interactive virtual classrooms using Learning Village technology offering distance learning to technical, trade and business schools in surrounding cities. With sustained leadership focus spanning nearly a decade, Naestved has become a model e-government.

Access or 'digital divide' issues are paramount issues for government leaders and in itself the question of the digital divide has many facets which include geographical, income, social, age, language and gender aspects. Governments need to understand the manifestations and implications of each within their particular jurisdictions and take corrective measures.

Infrastructure is perhaps the single most important overall e-community enabler for residents, businesses, healthcare facilities and educational institu-tions to thrive in a digital economy and society. As the next generation internet unfolds, rural communities, in particular, face significant access challenges. Like their small business counterparts, individual rural com-munities with small populations have little bargaining power with high-speed providers. Governments are exploring ways to facilitate aggregation of demand by region to attract providers. For example, Canada's Alberta province has embarked on a SuperNet project, a public/private partnership to extend high-speed access to the far corners of the province as part of a larger community and economic development strategy.

The Computer Systems Policy Project (CSPP) is a public policy advocacy group comprised of chairmen and chief executive officers from America's leading information technology companies. Their 'Readiness Guide for Living in the Networked World' is a self-assessment guide to assist commun-ities in achieving 'connectedness' in today's networked world (www.cspp.org). The CSPP characterises four stages of e-community development across a variety of criteria including network infrastructure (residential, commercial, wired/fixed/wireless, mobile wireless), access and applications (business, government, K-12, higher education, health, home), networked economy (innovation, workforce, consumer) and enablers (ubiquity, security, privacy, policy).

Milestone five: intergovernmental

The intergovernmental phenomenon is just beginning to emerge as a core ingredient of e-government. As boundaries of all sorts blur, those between and among governments are perhaps the 'fuzziest'. When this issue is discussed an anecdote from a family trip from Virginia to Florida with an unusually chatty pilot, comes to mind. For as the aeroplane flew down the east coast, the pilot would announce the flight's progress over each state along the way. Looking out the window, my 6-year-old son asked me 'How does he know? Where are the lines?' by which he meant the outlines of the states as they appear on a map. In many respects, the 'lines', just as on this aeroplane journey, are truly transparent. Physical world problems of disease, insects, global warming, terrorism and pollution know no boundaries. Couple this with technology that knows no boundaries and the effect on wider issues of governance is likely to be profound.

At the global level, quasi-governmental bodies are emerging to pool knowledge and resources to combat global problems. Within countries, there are growing needs to integrate national, state/provincial and local government operations, services and technologies. Citizens and businesses need to interact with all levels of government. Therefore, any robust e-government agenda must address intergovernmental linkages. Now is the time to launch the first pilots and begin meaningful intergovernmental deliberations around common processes and services. Within numerous states in the United States, such dialogue has already begun in the form of intergovernmental committees that meet to identify e-government opportunities, and address issues, infrastructure and integration. Some states offer city services on their websites. Others help the citizen or business navigate to the right place through personalisation techniques, such as zip code identifiers. Intergovernmental topics are on the conference agendas of nearly every national association. For example, in 2000, the National Association of State Information Resource Executives (NASIRE) held round-table discussions with representatives from other national associations serving municipal levels of government. Regardless of the government level, these initiatives need to be encouraged and supported with new funding mechanisms for intergovernmental initiatives.

The stakes inherent in intergovernmental integration include not only citizen convenience, but also leveraging business opportunities. As economic competition increases, reducing the time and financial burdens of complying with multiple levels of government regulation will be a distinct competitive advantage. The sheer weight of government can be lifted from businesses to make them faster to market, to open new international markets, and to enable higher performance in ongoing operations.

Milestone six: the policy environment

Creating a workable legal framework is another pillar of e-government success. Old laws have to change and new laws are needed. Perhaps even more importantly, legislative restraint is sometimes the best course of action in these still-early stages of a global networked economy. Members of oversight bodies need education and guidance on internet-related policy issues. A flurry of fundamental issues, including taxation, digital signatures, authentication, privacy, the digital divide, international trade, consumer protection, intellectual property rights, and telecommunications deregulation have appeared on the legislative agenda of virtually every country, state/ province and local governing body. Yet, a 1996 study commissioned by IBM's Institute for Electronic Government and conducted by the Strategic Computing and Telecommunications in the Public Sector programme at Harvard's John F. Kennedy School of Government found that fewer than 7 per cent of legislators felt personally knowledgeable to consider such decisions. Although this figure has undoubtedly improved since 1996, it remains a challenge and, in many cases, a barrier to progress.

National associations, public/private institutions, public policy organisations and think tanks have become core resources studying and advising law makers on policy issues. One successful model is the public–private United States internet Council (USIC) initiative. Funded by the private sector, the nonprofit USIC not only educates elected officials, but forms a network of legislators among the fifty US states to share model legislation and best practices. Specific committees and caucuses were established in state legislatures to be the centre of focus for all internet-related bills. Technology is no longer subjugated as an afterthought to a standing committee whose main purpose and member expertise is in some other domain. The USIC also bridges state legislatures with the United States Congress for inter-governmental coordination of internet-related legislation.

According to *E-Government: The Next American Revolution*, prepared by Hart-Teeter for the Council for Excellence in Government in September 2000, 66 per cent of Americans are concerned about the possibility of hackers breaking into government computers, making this the number one public concern about e-government. Fifty-three per cent are concerned about potential for less personal privacy. Clearly managing 'security' is a major challenge. However, even more important will be coming to grips with privacy policy issues and maintaining public trust. Workable solutions can be found. Poorly crafted privacy legislation will limit individual choice and restrict data flow that is critical to a robust information-based economy. Targeted privacy initiatives can preserve choice, boost consumer confidence and educate consumers.

Milestone seven: next generation internet

Milestone seven is the capstone of a competitive e-government strategy. It not only depends on progress toward other milestones, it is the one that will set governments apart in the future. Maintaining a focus on the horizon is a key challenge for public services, for if you define e-government in terms solely of today's environment, your government will never be a leader. High-speed connectivity is opening wide the doors to the next generation internet.

Imagine a billion people connected to the internet with the potential and dangers inherent in the scale and scope of their activities.

In this new environment, imagine a road crew in the field linked by video conference – on the screen of a handheld wireless device – both with the supervisor back in the government office and the contractor two states away. By streaming live video of the construction site and sharing engineering drawings, on-the-spot design changes can be made. Citizens will no longer just click on a form, rather they will click on an icon and a live government service representative will appear on the screen to help. This is the future of e-government.

Most people still confuse the internet with the world wide web. Today, 95 per cent of people view the web through their PC browsers. That will drop to just 40 per cent in the next 5 years. Japan is the first country to have broken through that barrier. By March 2000, more than 50 per cent of internet access in Japan was through devices other than the PC, including pagers, TVs, personal data assistants and telephones now acting as browsers.

The printing press cut the cost of information distribution by 99 per cent. Likewise, the internet cut the cost of disseminating information by 99 per cent. The next generation internet will do that again, it will cut the cost of information by a further 99 per cent. IBM's research team predicts a million-fold increase in the number of bytes of data available on the internet in the next 10 years. The pace of change is unlike anything we have encountered before and it is accelerating. The next generation internet is characterised by seven trends: fast, always on, everywhere, natural, intelligent, easy and trusted.

Fast

> Today, most users of the internet spend a large percentage of their time online waiting – waiting to get connected to a web site, waiting for pages to load, waiting for software to download. In contrast, the Next Generation internet (NGI) will provide the necessary speed – in other words, eliminate the World Wide Wait.
>
> (Patrick 2000)

It took approximately 15 years to increase bandwidth by a factor of ten yet, within the next 5 years, bandwidth will increase 150 times in capacity and speed. The quality of video over the internet will increase commensurately. Content management and distribution will be forever changed. When video over the internet is as common as email and as crisp as TV reception is today, a major shift in applications will occur. Nearly every agency of the City of Vancouver already has an impressive archive of video stored on their website – even pets up for adoption at the animal shelter! From its studio in Washington, DC, the Institute for Electronic Government website features an array of video talk shows, speakers and panels at national conferences, and mini-series on a variety of e-government topics.

To take one example, today, citizens must passively watch hours of scheduled televised legislative proceedings just to see one portion that may be of interest. Already technology exists whereby citizens can search and retrieve (or translate to text) just that portion of a video stored on a website that is of interest to them and simultaneously view related reference material. IBM's Cue Video, for example, uses not just voice recognition software, but also domain knowledge and machine learning to create a high-level search, browsing, and retrieval capability – of both text and visual objects.

Always on

Very soon there will be access to the internet without an elaborate dial-up or log-on sequence. Websites and applications will always be on, instead of vanishing and reappearing depending on network load. This means that citizens and businesses will have continuous instant access to you and your services – no matter where they are or what time of day.

This will affect how you staff your agencies, the definition of a work day and where you locate staff. Face to face will have a new meaning – it just will not be over a counter anymore. Face-to-face will be over internet video-conferencing. If your agency is not yet fully available 24 hours a day, 7 days a week, it will soon have to be.

Everywhere

Sooner than you may think, almost everything you purchase that's worth more than $10 or $20 – a refrigerator, a shirt, or a bicycle – will contain a tiny chip that can communicate via a wireless link to the internet. In such a world, connectivity is as common as air, and your watch, trees – even your dog – radiate data. Your watch could serve as a pager. Sensors on trees around your house could tell you – or your sprinkler – that the trees need watering. Your dog's collar could tell you where he is. Best of all, your lost car keys will be able to tell you where they are.

(Patrick 2000)

This is pervasive computing and it is a game-changing development. Computer scientists see it approaching a kind of mathematical extreme in which internet-connected, microscopic chips will literally disappear into all the things around us. The signs are already here. Today, the electronics of a car cost more that the mechanical parts. Most importantly of all, the scale and speed of such trends are growing all the time.

The New York State Division of Parole is already there. Using a small handheld device, parole officers can soon take pertinent information with them out into the field, and process information remotely. The information is accessible to the officers when and where they need it most, delivered in a way that is safe and convenient. Their hands are free. If you are a parole officer, that's important. Importantly, there is no laptop to carry around.

Natural

Today, people adapt to technology. We accept that it is often difficult to use. Soon, technology will adapt to people and become much more intuitive and easier to use. In many cases, you will not even realise you are using it. It will be natural. Technology will learn how to interact and adapt to you. The content available to us will become richer and more meaningful, and the delivery of that content will mirror much more closely the interactions that we experience in everyday life.

Human interactions, that have largely been missing from technology, will start to emerge. E-meetings, in which people communicate and share information through real-time video connections on the internet, are a good example. At IBM, e-meetings are becoming more and more frequent where employees can interact live, face-to-face with colleagues from around the world, and even share content – documents, spreadsheets, web-pages – in real time, while still honouring the very real need for security and privacy. In 2000, a worldwide e-meeting replaced a 4,000 person face-to-face meeting. The results received high marks on content delivery, convenience and education. Additionally, this approach saved over $3 million in cost avoidance.

Consider also the implications for computer-based training and distance learning. One of the biggest challenges of computer-based training is that the person who would normally tailor material to your needs, interests and abilities, the teacher, has been largely removed from the equation. Imagine if a computer 'teacher' could sense your boredom, either by a wandering mouse, or possibly even a reduced heart rate and speed up the material or make it more challenging? On the other side, what if the computer could 'see' the anxiety in your face, possibly by monitoring galvanic responses, and slow the material down, or go into a specific topic in more depth? The potential for successful models of distance learning will be leveraged with high-speed video capabilities, bringing the professor, classmates, and live class interactions, right to your screen in conjunction with course content and reference material.

Intelligent

In the not too distant future there will be an intelligent infrastructure, so that when I walk up to a device, it will register who I am, load my preferences, and customise the interface for me. It will be like walking up to a bank ATM and not having to tell it your language is English – or having to enter your PIN. It will already know that.

Today, information on the internet is largely unstructured. New standards are emerging for encoding web pages in a way that provides context to the pages. With that capability, web sites can begin to act on behalf of people to find solutions to problems. Organisations will be able to provide more targeted and higher quality services.

An intelligent infrastructure, coupled with increased computing power, will allow a much more personal vision of government to constituents. When a constituent interacts with an e-government, information that is relevant to them will be presented. The interface will be tailored to their needs and desires and it will be intelligent enough to bring things to their attention that they might find relevant.

The ability to capture and retrieve nontraditional types of information will also be increasingly important to governments as the baby-boomer generation begins to retire. As more and more employees leave the work-force, knowledge management will become critical in capturing expertise built up over the years as an organisational asset.

Easy

In the future, when we communicate or transact business using the internet, the whole experience will flow easily from one step to the next. Software and applications will be able to talk to one another and work across time and distance. There will be no need to re-enter data repeatedly or worry about formats or reboot because your Web browser caused your e-mail software to crash. The seamless integration of applications will enable us to get things done quickly, effectively, completely – and in the most productive way possible.

(Patrick 2000)

E-government is not just about creating portals. Complex legacy systems need to be modernised to take advantage of emerging technologies. Open standards and open systems will ensure that information flows seamlessly across departments and agencies – as well as up and down the jurisdictional chain.

Trusted

The internet is a public medium today, but will evolve into a public infrastructure serving public and private needs. These private needs will be met through enhanced understanding of personal preferences – even down to mood sensing and psychological profiling – and enhanced content delivery. The challenge is to protect both streams of data – personal collection and content delivery – over a public network.

Technology is rapidly moving toward finding solutions for security issues, ensuring that citizens identities can be unquestionably verified over the internet (through digital IDs), and that information that travels across networks can be secured beyond a reasonable doubt. Solutions for more complex issues associated with privacy, unfortunately, are lagging behind. When voice, video and alphanumeric data all travel over the network, every online transaction has privacy implications – rights, control over collection, dissemination and publication of personal data. The issue facing everyone and governments in particular, is trust. How do you establish not only security solutions, but also policy models that safeguard privacy as more and more information is collected and shared?

Conclusion

These seven milestones will take you to e-government, that much is guaranteed. However, this is not to underestimate the enormous leadership effort required. Consider the Commonwealth of Virginia and Naestved examples, much of their success is directly attributable to sustained leadership input over a 10-year period, spanning different political party administrations, and linked to this, substantial financial investments. Based upon analysis of the returns and rewards they are reaping today, it would appear to be a very small price to pay.

However, there is a need to be wary of shortcuts and detours. New entrants into the public sector marketplace will come and go over the long run. While trendy 'quick fixes' may be enticing, nothing replaces taking the future into your own hands with steadfast determination and specific goals. How fast you progress toward e-government is directly proportionate to funding. Solid business cases can be made for that investment. Also finding the right partner is critical. Governments face an almost insurmountable resource gap. Even the private sector faces a critical worldwide shortage of skilled resources. To expect to affordably 'own' the skilled resources needed to meet the coming challenges is simply unrealistic. In addition, governments cannot effectively keep pace with technological change and meet those challenges alone. Therefore, solid technology partners are essential if success is to be attained.

These are exciting times. With a little foresight, an aggressive approach toward each milestone, the right partner and perhaps even a little luck, e-government is within grasp.

References

Clift, S. (2000) *Top Ten E:democracy to Do List.* Online. Available HTTP: http:
www.e-democracy.org/do (8 December 2000)
Commonwealth of Virginia. (1999) *Economic Trends – First Quarter 1999.* Virginia:
Commonwealth Government.
Commonwealth of Virginia. (2000) *Technology in Virginia's Regions,* Virginia:
Commonwealth Government.

Government of Canada. (2000) *Smart Communities.* Online. Available HTTP: http: www.policyresearch.gc.ca (8 December 2000)

Hart, P. and Teete, B. (2000) *E:government: The Next American Revolution,* Washington: Council for Excellence in Government.

Patrick, J. (2000) *Measuring the Impact of the Next Generation internet,* Washington: IBM, Institute for Electronic Government.

Chapter 3

Centrelink, changing culture and expectations

Sue Vardon

Centrelink is the one-stop shop for many Australian Commonwealth government services. Now in operation for almost 4 years, it has evolved from a plan to integrate social security assistance and employment to a network of 1,000 sites of customer service centres, outreach services, agents and call centres providing a wide range of services on behalf of eleven Commonwealth and eleven state authorities. It employs 22,000 people and has 6 million customers spread the length and breadth of Australia. In the course of the evolution, there have been many changes to the way service offerings are tailored.

In the creation of Centrelink, the Commonwealth Government set some simple and clear objectives:

- Remove the complexity of government programmes for the customer
- Create a one-stop shop for citizens
- Introduce these services in the most efficient way, thereby providing savings to the government and the tax payer
- Maintain a high degree of accountability to government and hence the general public.

Centrelink was not the first attempt at creating a one-stop shop in Australia. The first serious attempt pre-Centrelink was the North-west One-stop shop Welfare centre (NOW) in the state of Victoria. This centre operated between July 1975 and the late 1980s. The model was developed based on co-location of the Commonwealth Department of Social Security, the Victorian Department of Social Welfare, local councils and representatives of voluntary agencies and community groups. The services provided included pensions and benefits, family assistance payments, supervision of probationers, parolees and wards, counselling, referral, information and interpreter services. It also provided a meeting place for user participation. Staff members from each separate agency carried out the respective functions side by side, rather than being trained to deliver all functions.

The eventual closure of the NOW centre was attributed to a number of factors including the lack of re-engineering of conflicting process of the respective agencies, withdrawal of political and agency support, issues of identity and organisational loyalty among staff members, wide differences in staff case loads and tensions over resources. Nevertheless, the community and customers responded positively to the NOW centre model and were more satisfied with the services they had received there than with the service ordinarily provided by the separate agencies (Wettenhall and Kimber 1996).

The rationale underpinning the creation of Centrelink

In 1991, the Australian Liberal and National Party coalition proposed to 'integrate the administration of payments and training functions by merging the Commonwealth Employment Service (CES) with the Department of Social Security (DSS) to created a more effective one-stop shop for unemployed persons' (Liberal and National Parties 1991). When they were elected to government in 1996, they delivered on this intention at the same time introducing a radical new model for job placement – the Job Network, a mix of public and private suppliers. Centrelink became the gateway to the job network and the place for all assessment for income security payments. Centrelink was instrumental in implementing the mutual obligation requirements of the new government.

Centrelink's brief was wider than simply employment services. The former Department of Social Security (now the Department of Family and Community Services) was charged by the Minister for Social Security, Senator Jocelyn Newman, with the task of streamlining five youth payments into one for young people and students. The resulting youth allowance was delivered by Centrelink and Centrelink took over child care payments a few months later.

At the launch of Centrelink in September 1997, the prime minister, the Hon John Howard said:

> From the moment I entered Parliament in 1974 and began talking to constituents about their various problems, I began hearing complaints about the number of agencies you had to visit. And what focused my mind at the time was that so many people felt that if only they could go to one place and have all their business done in that one spot it would be a lot more efficient, it would be a lot more human and it would make a great deal more sense. The consolidation in Centrelink of so many of the services of the government that interact with people will provide, of course a more human face and a more efficient service. In the past we have encouraged people to go from one location to another and we have often confused them with a lot of administrative duplication. And in one very big stroke Centrelink cuts through that duplication. Centrelink

consolidates in an efficient modern fashion the major service delivery activities of the federal government.

(Howard 1997)

The Minister for Social Security (and Centrelink) Senator, the Honourable Jocelyn Newman also said in a speech at the time of the agency's launch:

The agency will bring together several areas of Commonwealth service delivery into a one-stop shop for a range of government services. Service delivery agencies have been established overseas notably in the UK and New Zealand but the new agency takes the concept of a single-point government service delivery further. Unlike overseas counterparts, the agency will not operate solely as an administrative entity within a department of state or be limited to single portfolio responsibilities. . . . The agency's customers will have a single point of contact – a one-stop shop – for a range of government services.

(Newman 1997)

Centrelink was created from a political agenda to take hold of the complexity of the way bureaucracies had organised themselves to deliver services and to change the face of government in a radical way. The complexity was placed behind the counter and the public service was challenged to reshape the way that they implemented government policy.

Instead of one department being given responsibilities for integrated services, the government decided to create an independent statutory authority to be a provider for many policy departments using business partnership agreements. Legislation was enacted to create the Commonwealth Services Delivery Agency in 1997. The government introduced a predominantly private sector board whose challenge was to bring the best of the private sector practices together with the best of the public service practices. The changes caused a cascade of improvement in customer service; outcome/output definition; transparency of costs and performance measures that made sense. There was an expectation that the removal of overheads would deliver significant savings to government. A special efficiency dividend of 10 per cent to be returned over 3 years was placed on the new agency. To date these efficiencies have been delivered.

The Commonwealth Services Delivery Agency became Centrelink. There was a search for a name that was friendly, did not have bureaucratic overtones and could not be turned into initials nor would it limit the scope to welfare alone. It should not infer the superiority of government as a supplier, but as a partner with the community and customers. There was extensive customer research to find the word to project these images. Two thousand suggestions from staff were also considered. 'Centrelink' seemed to satisfy all expectations.

Centrelink has passed through many phases in its pursuit of the prime minister's and Minister for Family and Community Service's aspirations. There are probably four overlapping phases that can be identified so far with plans in place for future directions.

Phase 1: the creation of the one-stop shop

Centrelink was built from the two networks of the Department of Social Security and parts of the Department of Employment, Education, Training and Youth Affairs (Figure 3.1). Each had been in existence for decades and had developed quite different cultures. The social security culture was process based and controlled by tight rules of necessity to ensure that people received their correct entitlements and no more. They had introduced a customer service focus but the delivery of a payment was an end in itself for most people. Staff from Employment, Education and Youth Affairs were outcome focused. Job seekers were to be found work and students helped into an education opportunity. They were supported by guidelines and programme funds which gave a fair degree of creative opportunity for staff to tailor a solution according to the circumstances. Both groups of staff were strongly influenced at a personal level to come to work to make a difference and to 'help people'.

Those of us who were building Centrelink wanted to capture the best of both these cultures at the same time to set a special identity for the new agency (Figure 3.2). We identified those characteristics that would define our place and purpose. We created our own shared behaviours – listening, respecting, finding solutions, behaving with integrity and exploring. From the beginning we were mindful that the ministers wanted better experiences for the citizen with government so we made customer service a prime focus for our reforms. The biggest cultural shift for everyone was to become performance-focused as we were funded through business partnership agreements and had to satisfy regularly measured key performance indicators. A balanced score card was introduced to emphasise this performance focused approach. The Kaplan and Norton model for developing such a scorecard approach was used. (Kaplan and Norton 1993). Key performance areas were determined for each of Centrelink's five corporate goals and an emphasis was placed upon achieving vertical integration of the scorecard throughout the organisation. Disparate performance data sources were brought together into one central assessment point and presented as green (met) and yellow (unmet) dots. Identifying and developing robust measurements which would serve to drive forward the goal of performance improvement, particularly in respect of defining metrics for those areas traditionally hard to capture into substantive data, took many months.

A campaign of listening to customers started immediately. In the first 2 years we listened to around 9,500 customers in small, specific feedback

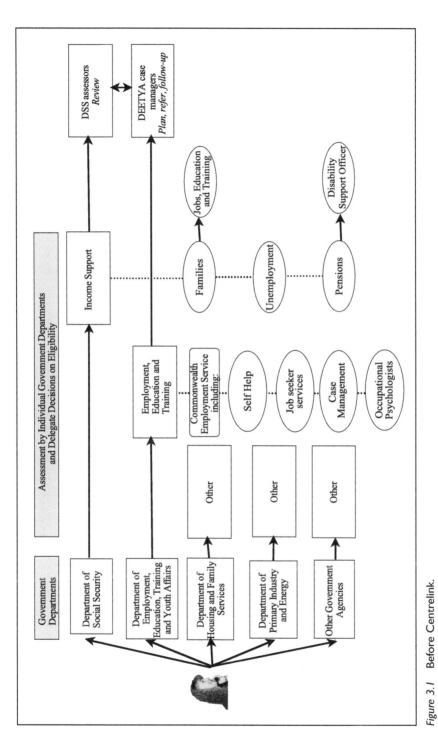

Figure 3.1 Before Centrelink.

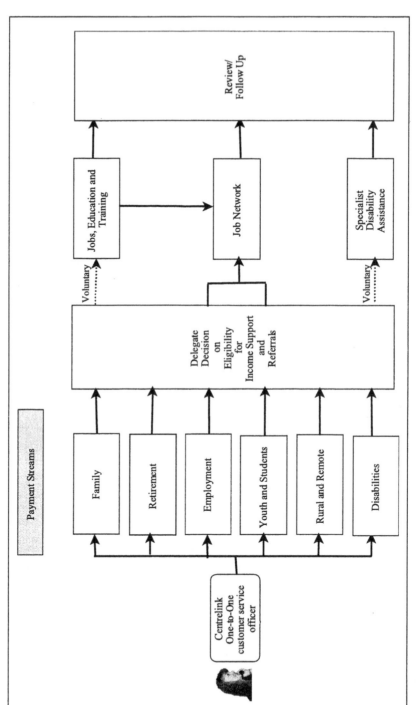

Payment Streams

Centrelink One-to-One customer service officer

Family

Retirement

Employment

Youth and Students

Rural and Remote

Disabilities

Delegate Decision on Eligibility for Income Support and Referrals

Voluntary

Voluntary

Jobs, Education and Training

Job Network

Specialist Disability Assistance

Review/ Follow Up

Figure 3.2 Centrelink, the one-stop shop.

workshops with Centrelink staff. These workshops were held at the local level usually in non-Centrelink sites. Twenty-three were run in five of our customers' languages other than English. We learned that customers do not care which departments had responsibility for providing for their needs; they did not care what the products were called; few knew the difference between the three tiers of government. They did care though about being able to tell their circumstances only once and being dealt with by a caring person. They wanted simplicity, accuracy and friendly service. These standards became our benchmarks for service improvement.

The staff who were listening were surprised by some of the feedback and often made immediate improvements to their local office. On one occasion the feedback was that the sign saying 'We reserve the right to call the police if your behaviour is offensive' made them feel like criminals. The sign had been placed up to warn a few people, but the effect had been generalised. The sign was immediately taken down. On another occasion, customers asked why a computer could not be made available for them to do their resumés. A computer was installed in the office the next day and the facility is now available widely throughout the Centrelink network.

The look and feel of Centrelink offices started to change dramatically. Out went the forbidding counters to be replaced by brightly coloured, open-plan offices and plants. Many more points of service for interviews were opened by bringing the back office people forward to the frontline. This did not suit some staff who had spent many years effectively trying to escape from face to face interviews. Service by appointment started and customer liaison officers walked the queues to help people who only wanted information or to hand in a form. Queue management became a priority and the length of time people waited was reduced in most places. Customer service training was introduced and customer service champions were trained. Name tags for all staff including the chief executive officer are required to be worn.

The emphasis on customer service raised a few concerns. There was a fear that by taking this approach, there would be a temptation to make a positive decision even if there was not an entitlement. We went on a campaign that good customer service is accurate customer service. There were those who argued that the ministers or the contracting departments were the customers. Recognising the many equal stakeholders, the departments are referred to as clients. There were those who said that customer was a word connected to choice and many of the people we assisted were not necessarily there by choice. We took a broader definition of the word. In the end, we refer to the customer by name when we assist them so we try not to get caught up in semantics. We customise our language for the client departments and refer to 'veterans' and 'job seekers'.

The newly created Centrelink presented a single front for government, but internally service is still provided in silos. There are families teams, employment teams, youth teams, retirement and disabilities teams. Reinforcing this, we badged the organisations in the front office by service type. Retired customers like to be dealt with away from the queues of job seekers. Some of our offices have contracts with the Department of Veterans, Affairs and we have specially designated areas for this service with staff specially trained to bring together all the veterans services in one area. There are specially designated areas for job seekers to access self-help touch screens for job search and special computers to write resumés and phones to ring potential employers.

This streaming whilst undoubtedly an advance, still does not totally satisfy the expectation that a person with complex issues across streams, stays still and has a holistic service. Individual customers still have to move between streams and teams, to some extent.

We widened the methods of service delivery to include education seminars and job expos. There was an encouragement to reach out to communities to work with other agencies in finding broader more systemic and more creative solutions to problems.

As Centrelink opened, so did its opportunities. The government had a face and a network throughout Australia to which it could attach further services. We took stock of our capabilities. These included expertise in high volumes of payments; a network outreaching to the whole of Australia; a customer service approach; call centres; a capacity to implement major policy change fairly rapidly and connection to local communities. We offered these to other departments. A small isolated service, the Tasmanian Freight Equalisation Scheme, was attached to this larger body, giving its staff an opportunity to have a career in a larger organisation. The Government Information Service in Tasmania was introduced using the capacity of the call network.

The Government also responded to the rural people's desire for special-ised services by opening two rural call centres using the Centrelink call centre network. Three indigenous call centres were established so that indigenous Australians could speak with their own people. Centrelink bid for and won a contract to be the call centre for passports. In addition, Centre-link now delivers many services to farmers as part of the government's policy response to agriculture issues.

The range of the client departments now includes:

- Family and Community Services
- Transport and Regional Services
- Employment, Workplace Relation and Small Business
- Education, Training and Youth Affairs
- Health and Aged Care
- Agriculture, Fisheries and Forestry
- Veterans' Affairs

- Foreign Affairs and Trade
- Immigration and Multicultural Affairs
- State housing authorities.

However, whilst Centrelink has been chosen as the preferred supplier for the social security system and the gateway to reform in employment, the rest of its work is based on competitive tendering or presentation of a business case to bid for new business. We had to develop business acumen to understand our costs and to understand how to run a business, rather than a traditional bureaucracy. The staff of Centrelink constantly present us with ideas for new business offerings.

The Centrelink network is a convenient place in which to outpost other government services such as the Child Support Agency and in twenty-one sites around Australia people can resolve issues about child maintenance and child payments in one place. When the government recently introduced a new tax system, it introduced choice to citizens in payments and Centrelink is one of three agencies providing the Family Assistance Office.

There has been some concern in Australia that services are disappearing from remote and rural Australia. To address this concern, the Commonwealth government, in conjunction with local councils and communities, has opened Rural Transaction Services (RTCs) in some towns with populations of less than 3,000 people. These provide services such as basic personal banking, phone, fax, post and Medicare Easyclaim. Centrelink has been working closely with the councils of these communities to ensure that the Centrelink services delivered from the RTCs meet the needs of the particular community. The services are generally self-help facilities with access to a range of Centrelink forms and information material, a telephone service with lines dedicated to Centrelink Call and a form's lodgement facility. Staff of the RTCs are trained to respond to basic Centrelink enquiries.

Other governments

We are experimenting with offering our sites to state governments particularly in rural and remote parts of Australia where it is more cost efficient for a single state officer to deliver services surrounded by a team of colleagues from another agency, who can assist with appointments and backup. In Singleton, a rural town in New South Wales, the state government housing department official is co-located with Centrelink. This is safer for the staff person and our customers who have public housing issues can get service from just one office.

Most state governments in Australia are looking at some form of one-stop shop. In Tasmania, Centrelink and Service Tasmania (the state government one-stop shop) established a partnership under which the two organisations would work together to pilot delivery of both Commonwealth and state government service to the community from a number of common sites. This is being enhanced by the Trials of Innovative Government Electronic Regional Services (TIGERS) project. This offers a unique opportunity to model and pilot the integration of services across three tiers of government. Centrelink sites will deliver selected over-the-counter services on behalf of all three jurisdictions and will offer online service based on life events which can then be forwarded to relevant organisations on behalf of the customer. It will extend the Centrelink-operated Government Information Call Centre to answer queries for all tiers of government.

In Western Australia a very large state with small towns separated by huge geographical distances, the state government has created 76 telecentres to operated as one-stop shops for three tiers of government in remote areas. They act as agents for Centrelink services.

Phase 2: a new service delivery model

Once the physical changes had happened to create Centrelink, there was an opportunity to extract greater value from the consolidation of services and to move up the knowledge value chain. After 12 months in operation, Centrelink undertook an organisational review that examined the lessons learned from customers and staff and looked at a range of performance issues across all aspects of the business: in other words how was the current model of service delivery shaping up? Continuing to listen to customers through value creation workshops, we reflected on what people actually expected from government and an understanding of the way their experience brought them to government.

We were constantly reminded that people came for help when they were experiencing an event in their life. We announced a new approach to service delivery (Figue 3.3) that has as its cornerstone a 'life events' approach. The life events approach is a new construct for the delivery of government services. It is an approach based on the experiences of people in the community rather than the payments, services or programmes devised by government departments. We needed to tip the bureaucracy upside down to present an approach to service delivery from the customer's point of view. Service based on life events is more intuitive, logical and immediately recognisable for customers.

Customers will be able to approach Centrelink and describe their individual circumstances and the particular life event(s) they are experiencing and in return they will receive a personalised solution containing the products and services that meet their needs and obligations. In this way, Centrelink will deliver to customers, service offers tailored to their particular situation and customers will no longer have to know the right questions to ask to gain access to all of their entitlements. Increasingly it will be the task of Centre-link, not the customer, to sort out the complexities of government.

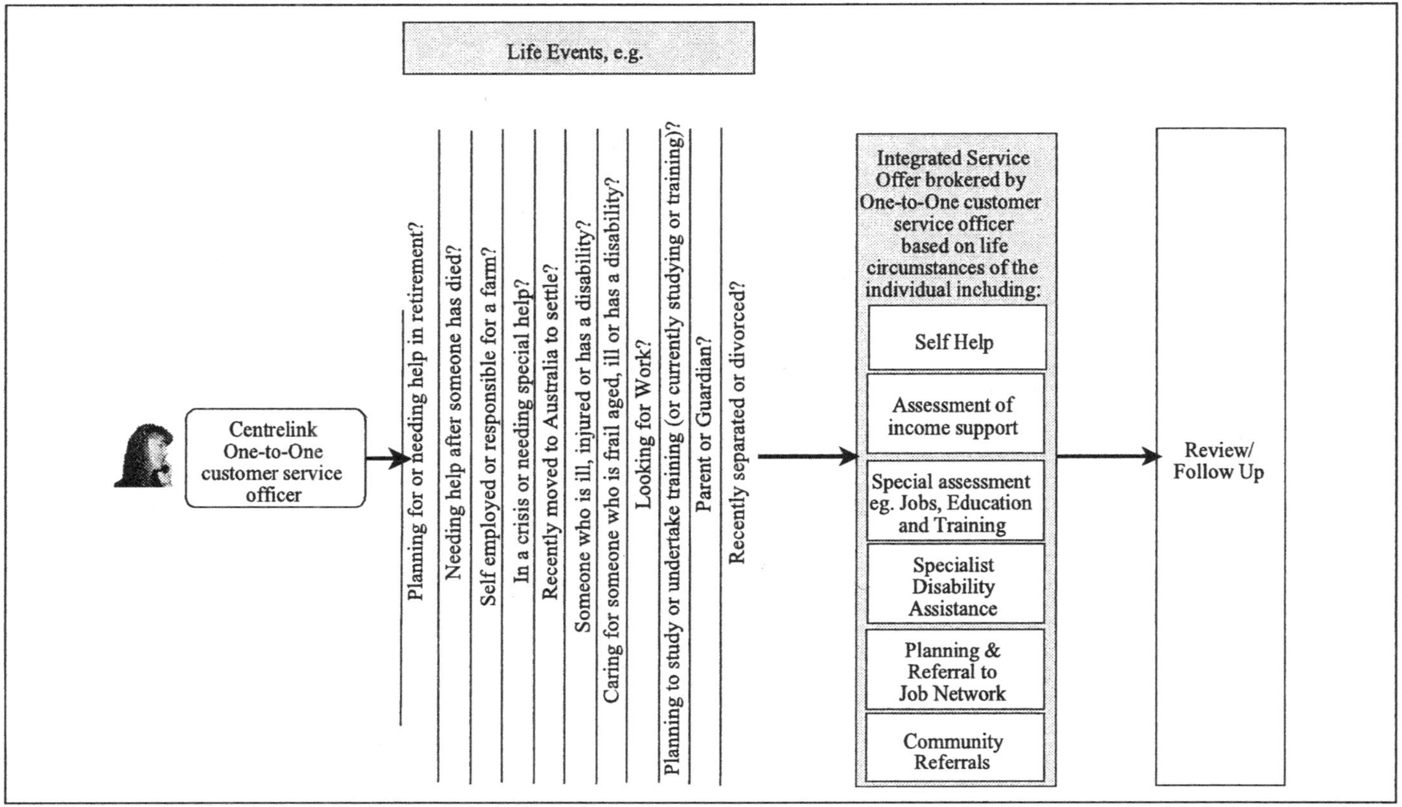

Figure 3.3 Centrelink, the new service delivery model.

This approach will enable Centrelink to deliver further on the Government's promise for a one-stop shop that would be easier to access and more responsive.

In mapping a life events approach, we identified eleven reasons for people coming to us:

- Planning for or needing help in retirement
- Parent or guardian
- Recently separated or divorced
- Needing help after someone has died
- Someone who is ill, injured or has a disability
- Caring for someone who is frail aged, ill or has a disability
- Recently moved to Australia to settle
- Looking for work
- Self-employed or responsible for a farm
- In a crisis situation or needing special help
- Planning to study or undertake training (or currently studying or training).

Taking on particular life event, for example, 'Are you planning for or needing help in retirement?', we can map the various products and services that we deliver on behalf of a number of our client departments (Figure 3.4).

We are redesigning all the literature of our organisation such as newsletters, forms and publicity to reflect the life events approach. Our most recent publication, 'What to do if someone dies', brings together information from Centrelink, the Department of Veterans' Affairs, the Department for Family and Community Services, and the Consumer Affairs Division of the Treasury. Our web site has taken on the life events frontage. We are working with the Office of Government On Line to connect our web site to a broader Access Australia portal.

We introduced the one main contact model or the one-to-one officer as we call it. Even though Centrelink commenced life as a convenient place for many types of government business, we still had not solved the problem of the customer having to tell their story once only, nor being able to provide the caring face of someone who knew them. With six million customers, this was a challenge. One of our offices took up that challenge and allocated pools of customers to each customer service office with the name of the officer was attached to the electronic record. This approach worked and it has spread. However, it is also clear that not every service customer wants a personal officer and a significant proportion prefer to conduct their business with us via the call centres. However, those that do opt for the more personalised approach can make appointments via a special call centre line. A collateral benefit for the organisation was that work was now more evenly spread and the good performers are not covering for those who were working less efficiently.

Centrelink One-to-One customer service officer

Life Event: Are you planning for or needing help in retirement?

Integrated Service Offer brokered by One-to-One customer service officer based on the life circumstances of the individual including:

How to claim

Possible payments and products	Claim forms to issue	Information to request	Associated Products	Internal referrals, services and information provision including: Social workers, Financial Information services Officers, Jobs, Education and Training Advisors, Multicultural Service Officers, Interpreter Services, Indigenous Specialist Officers, Centrelink Community Officers, Rural Officers, Rent Dedcution Scheme, Assurance of Support Unit	External referrals, services and information provision including: Centrelink agents, Community Agent Program, Veteran's Information, Income assessment for residential aged care fees, Hearing services, Assurance of Support, Claiming overseas pension entitlements
Age Pension	Claim for Pension	consider payment for partner	Overseas pensions, income assessment for aged care residence		
Pension Bonus Scheme	Pension Bonus Scheme Registration	current employment details			
Commonwealth Seniors Health Card	Commonwealth Seniors Health Card Claim	latest available tax noticeof assessment			
Widow Allowance	Claim for Widow Allowance	proof of widow status	Centrepay		
Special Benefit	Claim for Special Benefit	proof of hardship	Centrepay		
Retirement Assistance for Farmers Scheme	Farm Details Form(with other payment claim form)	title deed of farm property, legal transfer document of farming assets			
	in addition to proof of identity, tax file number, proof of age, residency, income/assests		supplementary payments may include rent assistance, telephone allowance, pharmaceutical alloance, mobility allowance etc		

Figure 3.4 Life event map.

Results from the first stage of implementation of one-to-one arrangements in our customer service network indicate that:

- Customers are pleased with the more holistic, individual service and as a result are more confident in the decisions made about their entitlements.
- Staff are enjoying the increased control they have over their everyday work and report greater job satisfaction.
- Efficiency dividends are being realised with decisions being made more quickly, arrears being maintained at low levels, customer traffic being reduced and the number of reviews and appeals of decisions being lower in number.

That part of Centrelink's work that provides the social security payments is regulated by over 80,000 rules. Even when people specialise in an area, it is complex and ever changing. In response to this, we are designing smart decision support systems that will assist our staff in delivering accurate and appropriate service offers to customers. These systems mirror the logic a human expert uses to arrive at a decision. A smart system guides staff through the necessary policy rules and legislation. The use of such support happens during the interview as the staff member enters the customer's information into the system. We have introduced a version of this in employment services and a full version relating to families' payments and services was released at the end of 2000.

Smart systems also have a 'what if' capability that enables the customer to test a number of scenarios to assess the impact of possible changes in their circumstances. This approach means customers do not have to fill out forms and they do not have to know precisely for what they might be eligible. It also ensures more accurate and consistent decision-making and provides a tailored service. When an early version of the families smart system was tested, there was greater confidence from the customers that they were getting a free and accurate service. The fact that the legislation was shown on the screen at the same time, provided certainty that they were getting a fair deal.

We have built an electronic reference suite of all the guidelines, rules and policy interpretations that we are obliged to follow. Although a great improvement on previous information manuals which were typically poorly updated, it is still a challenge to find all the complex information that governs all Centrelink practices. Thus, we are currently building an advanced search capacity into this tool and anticipate good levels of response to this from both staff and customers alike.

Perhaps one of the most interesting developments arising out of the use of technology has been the introduction of the Centrelink Education Network. It is a challenge to get good information, particularly technical information, to staff all over Australia quickly. The Ford company had solved the problem with Fordstar, a satellite-based training platform that allowed interactive learning direct to Ford distributors. Learning from this model we built three classrooms in Canberra that connect via satellite to most Centrelink sites. Subject experts make presentations from the classroom and staff watch on television, connected to a call-in service for questions and can answer questions via a touch pad.

Phase 3: enhancing the one-stop shop

Having spent 2 years working with the tools and rules given to us by departments we stood back and reflected about how we could be more valued to government and citizens. We were still, in practice, administering silos albeit more sensitively. The processes differed according to each department and often were different within the same department. We had too many access points for departmental officials to send in instructions, often without a clear understanding of who was going to pay for the initiatives and the demands on some parts of our organisation, particularly the knowledge team who were responsible for reporting statistically, were great. Priority setting was a challenge. There was duplication in our own organisation and inconsistency in how things were done and the style in which they were done. We needed to coordinate workflows better and im-prove the speed to market for new initiatives. Governments like their policies implemented quickly and we still had cumbersome systems which provided a very real barrier to achieving change quickly.

Within this context we looked at the customer in/customer out chain of service delivery (Figure 3.5) and realised that there were four main processes:

* Accessing Centrelink (initial contact with the customer)
* Assessment of need and entitlement and obligation
* Plan development and referral
* Ongoing contact

We separated out two functions: (1) negotiation with the client depart-ments and (2) building the core processes.

Negotiation with the client departments became the province of the national managers of community segments – families, rural and housing, employment service, disability and carers, multicultural, youth and students, retirement, indigenous and international. This was our way of providing the client departments with designated senior officers to negotiate business requirements, business pricing and any concerns they had with us. For us it meant narrowing the front and forcing priorities to be set. The design of the core processes was handed to the Service Integration Shop, which is now testing simplification and re-engineering processes throughout our whole of government service delivery responsibility. We have been impressed with the

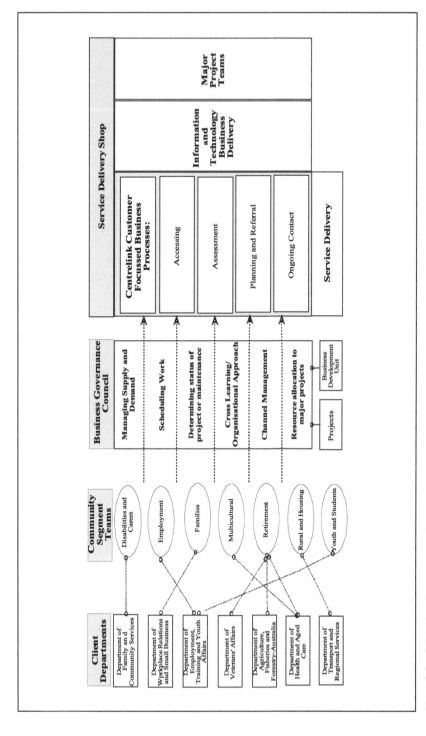

Figure 3.5 Enhancing the one-stop shop.

thought that two-thirds of all process is not value added and making inroads into reducing this figure represents a key challenge.

At the same time the information and technology (I and T) area was redesigned to create a one business approach (see Treadwell 2000). Previously the I and T group was structured in a traditional hierarchical way with clear stovepipes and individual responsibility and accountability held by various managers. This model did not allow the flexibility or responsiveness that would be required in coming years and was not sufficiently collaborative. There were also difficulties in managing supply and demand across the group and aligning to business need.

The new model is based on providing a single entry point to I and T and constructing how we run our business on the continuum of the end-to-end business process. This has allowed a better alignment to the business and given business an easier way of dealing with I and T. Business is now better placed to articulate its requirements and I and T is more effective at providing solutions sourced internally or externally and giving better value for money.

The I and T group set new goals based on its twin objectives of 'Delivering today; transforming tomorrow'. The goals they set are:

- *Capability to do the expected:* to meet business demand and maintain business operations rations.
- *Seamless change:* to undertake all I and T work with minimal disruption to users and customer.
- *Efficient business:* to provide value for money to Centrelink, our business clients and the community through efficient I and T operations and effective I and T solutions.
- *Excelling I and T people:* to recruit, develop and support I and T people in a way that enable them to excel in their contributions to Centrelink.
- *Information as an asset:* to provide Centrelink with superior intellectual capital through data integrity, data processing and knowledge solutions.
- *Boundary free:* to ensure I and T is sufficiently open and agile to enable Centrelink to undertake any business.

There are four quadrants of work which the I and T group presently supports and is building the foundations for the change programme for the future.

Customised services

The present service delivery network of mobile workers, customer service centres, call centres, shop fronts and agents, is spread across a land mass of 7,692,030 square kilometres. This is thirty-two times the size of the United Kingdom. We deliver seventy different products and services; send over 100 million letters and answer 20 million incoming calls; process 3.2 billion customer-related transactions per year and offer on-line access to job seeking. The 22,000 users plough through more than 10 million computer screens per day.

To support this, our technology platform processes 11 million transactions per day (400 per second). Our applications staff have built and change regularly, 11 million lines of code. The system is available more than 99.9 per cent during business hours. The mainframe capacity is 5,500 MIPS and we have 15 terabytes of disk storage and 200 terabytes of tape storage. The I and T people have built a satellite-based remote access lap top capability that can access the mainframe in the remotest parts of Australia.

The corporate intranet, Centrenet, was established in 1998, to deliver information and interactive services to our staff throughout Australia. The scale of Centrenet makes it one of the largest public or private intranets deployed in Australia. Centrenet set out with five major principles that have defined its evolution. These principles are:

- Decentralised content development to avoid workflow bottlenecks
- Compliance with the World Wide Web Consortium (WC3) standards to maximise portability flexibility and choice of internet best practice in the future
- Recognition that Centrenet provides not just electronic publishing, but a complete service delivery environment, offering extensive opportunities and capabilities for staff and the public
- Recognition that Centrenet represents an organisation learning opportunity, maximising the number of staff who can understand the capabilities and opportunities of the internet technologies that underpin Centrelink's future electronic service delivery strategy
- Recognition that Centrenet provides a migration platform where direct customer service ideas can be developed and test internally, or with staff assisting, the customer before being deployed directly and independently to the customer.

Centrenet provides an online phone book; entitlement ready reckoners; people management interrogation tools including employment/pay self services; ideas laboratories; the reference suite of rules; rumour confirmation or rejection and a wealth of information about our products and services and the teams within Centrelink who provide these services. Some other departments with whom we do business are provided with access to the Centrenet via a newly developed extranet to enable them to make use of assessment tools.

We trialled a web post office for the youth allowance customer by delivering letters using the internet and world wide web as the delivery mechanism. The trial was discontinued when the customer group became frustrated that it was only a one-way service and they were not able to reply via the net. We still need to solve the problems of authentication before we can advance this option.

Indirect services

We bulk 232 million payments a year electronically through 350 financial institutions into individual customer accounts. We have developed a facility called Centrepay, where a customer can elect to have deductions made from an income security payments for essential bills like housing or those payments which sustain a secure living environment. This has been so successful that we are scaling it up to provide a wider range of payments in the customer's interest. The housing authorities are pleased to receive regular payments as well for the deduction of a small fee.

Business to business

All government agencies in Australia are building business to business capability and Centrelink is no exception. Centrelink transmits customer data electronically to client departments, to allow referrals to occur. We accept data from other agencies and use it in data matching to identify potential cases of fraud. We have plans in place to improve our purchasing by using electronic procurement.

There are still issues associated with privacy and security of sensitive data transmitted over public networks, such as the internet. We will not progress our electronic agenda in e-business until we are satisfied that these concerns have been addressed.

Customer self-service

There are 300 touch screen kiosks in Centrelink customer services offices that provide an up-to-date access to a huge job vacancy data base called Australian Job Search, a product maintained by the Department of Employment, Workplace Relations and Small Business. These touch screens are very popular and are supported in our offices by telephones that can be used by job seekers to ring potential employers or job network members.

A customer self-service telephone facility to provide payment details was introduced for 3,000 customers in a trial in 1999. This resulted in improvements to customer service, but also provided important information about usage patterns, privacy and security issues as a precursor to future developments.

Phase 4: the future model

The key elements of service in 2005 for Centrelink customers will be access, choice, value, integration, connecting and brokering (Figure 3.6). Much of

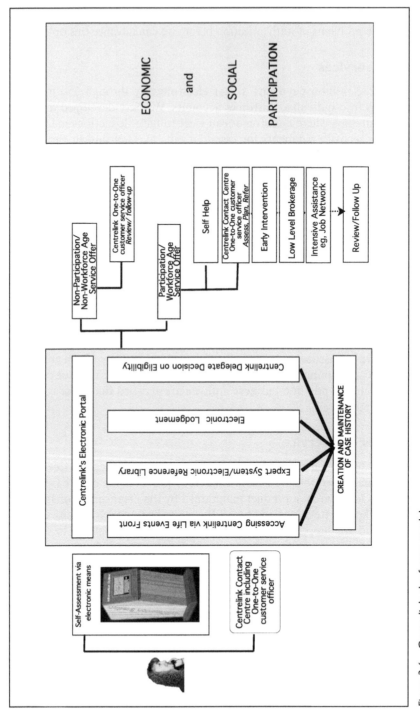

Figure 3.6 Centrelink, the future model.

how we will provide these services will be based on the use of technology. One of the key differences is the connectivity to a full range of service provided and brokered by Centrelink, applicable to the individual's circumstances. Our advanced customer relationship management skills will allow us to know intimately, the needs and preferences of each individual customer and our expert systems will allow them to make many choices themselves. Many of our customers will never need to visit an office or talk to our staff. All their interactions will be online if they choose.

We will operate as a value network, having established partnerships and alliances with a range of providers in the human services sector and will have extended our reach into associated industries. As an example, the job seeker will:

- Be able to contact Centrelink using multiple technical, virtual and personal channels.
- Determine their own eligibility for a range of payments and services.
- Negotiate a preparing for work contract with Centrelink, based on their mutual obligation to seek work whilst receiving employment support.
- Connect with a private sector job network provider to find employment.
- Organise his/her banking and financial arrangements through us online.
- Be referred in real time through shared appointment systems to companies who help job seekers put together resumés, provide career and training advice and help them obtain the 'look' they want for their interview.
- Connect and interact with a range of relevant organisations such as transport, health, housing, social activities and groups of common interests.
- Have their choice, selections and referral kept up to date in our databases to enable us to target our information and presentation to their preferences.

Our present model is based on the general customer and our response is individualised when they approach us. The future model looks to the profiled customer and a greater understanding of different customer groups, so that we can streamline and outreach and anticipate based on what we know of general characteristics of a subset of the population.

Our present model does not differentiate between channels. People contact us by whatever means are available using all channels. One-to-one service is at the most expensive end of the range and we want to develop it for people who need intensive help. There is no need, however, to provide it for students who have indicated they would prefer to do business electronically and for the government, cheaply. We need to understand our channels better – mail, call centres, electronic service delivery, and one-to-one service. We have begun a modelling exercise in conjunction with an external agency to identify and understand the mix and use of service access channels for the future to provide a 'what if' capability to assess future property and staffing requirement at both the macro and local level. This work is establishing a base year by determining current usage of access channels and projecting this forward 5 years using a range of known or assumed variables, such as changing population and customer base; new channel capability (such as self service pay details through Interactive Voice Response) and changes in Centrelink's service offerings taking a particular note of client department specifications and anticipated customer behaviour.

We will always provide a human service in Centrelink. There is concern in the community that we will participate in increasing the divide between information-rich and information-poor communities. We are continually restating that information technology provides freedom to deliver holistic services more comprehensively and for some the self-help capacity will be a choice. For those who do not make that choice, we will be there for them in offices, in outreach services and on the phone.

Our present model offers standard business hours that are about to be extended to 8.00 a.m.–5.00 p.m. We do open late at night and Saturday's when peak loads occur, but this is the exception. Our families call line is open from 8.00 a.m. to 8.00 p.m. Our future model is a 24 hour service delivery, 7 days a week. We will use technology to enable us to provide these extended services.

Our present model has us internally connected and integrated using the life events model and we have information technology connections to those client departments with whom we do present business. Our future model based on open systems will open our smart decision systems to enable data entry; electronic lodgement of forms and 'what if' testing by others. The personal file will of course be protected and only accessed by authorised, authenticated customers. We will connect via our web site to all other governments using the life events framework, so that all levels of government can make their offerings available in one place.

Our present model has limited agents who act on our behalf. The future model identifies that there will be many more agents. We see a growth in call centres and a change to customer contact centres, as they provide service via internet channels as well. We are not rushing into internet service on a personal level because our experience in opening new channels indicates that there will only be an increase in demand and no reduction on other channels. This is very costly. We are focusing on self-help via the internet as a preferred option but it will be difficult to hold back the tide of demand. Already we have two call centres answering internet queries, but because of problems of authentication we can only reply in general terms or over the phone for personal information.

Our present model has a moderate use of e-business. Our future model will capitalise on e-business in the four quadrants described above.

Our present model offers mainly Commonwealth services and some state housing services. Our future model envisages value-added offers based on life events, for example. If an outreach worker visits an older person to answer questions about a pension, the mobile lap top will access other parts of government and we can do other business for them while we are there.

Our present model is a fairly basic offering of standard services to client departments. Our future model after our process redesign, will enable us to analyse an outcome they wish to see and provide them with more than one suggestion about how it could be best achieved with differentiated channels and costing proposals.

Our present model still requires specialisation internally because of the complexities of all the business we do. Our future model will allow one officer to access the range of services electronically using smart systems and an e-reference suite.

Conclusion

In our first 18 months, a new agency was created with an emphasis on physical changes whilst reform in both social security and employment policies were introduced. There was pressure to deliver a financial dividend, as well as service improvement and increased productivity. We have reduced the cost of service to departments by approximately 20 per cent. In the second 18 months, we found ways to respond more intuitively to customer circumstances and to find the opportunities to streamline government by identifying core processes and applying them to all our client departments' work. When this is completed, we will have made headway into making government simpler.

It is recognised that the business of government is too complex for Centrelink to be a one-stop shop in all cases for all its customers, but it aims to provide a 'whole of government' approach to service delivery enabling customers to get most of the information, services and solutions they need from the Commonwealth in one place. Further, the one-stop shop concept has the power to unite all levels of government in co-operation. All levels of government aspire in their service delivery visions to make government access simpler and easier. The people of Australia have problems reconciling and differentiating levels of government. The story of Centrelink is not just about uniting Commonwealth Government services but how, by creative use of location and technology, we can carry each other's brands and services through shared channels. This is the greatest service delivery challenge.

Acknowledgements

The author wishes to acknowledge the many unpublished papers and submissions written by Centrelink staff from which was drawn the information for this chapter. The figures contained within this chapter were prepared by Louis Chan and Nikki Tran.

References

Kaplan, R. and Norton, D. (1993) 'Putting the balanced scorecard to work', *Harvard Business Review* September-October: 134–47.

Liberal and National Parties. (1991) *Fightback! Taxation and Expenditure Reform for Jobs and Growth,* Canberra: Liberal and National Parties.

Newman, J. (1997) 'Achieving Excellence in service delivery – changing service delivery arrangements for the Commonwealth Government'. Opening address AIC Conference Service Delivery in the Public Sector

Treadwell, J. (2000) 'Serving Australia on land and online', Canberra: Centrelink (unpublished).

Wettenhall, R. and Kimber, M. (1996) 'One-stop-shopping: Notes on the concept and some Australian Initiatives', Public Sector Papers 2/96, Canberra: Centre for Research in Public Sector Management, University of Canberra.

Chapter 4

Brisbane

A reflection on a journey

Judith Dionysius

Situated on the eastern seaboard of the Australian continent, Brisbane was officially declared a city in 1902 following the opening of the area to free settlement in 1842. The City of Brisbane Act (1924) created a city government to carry out the functions previously performed by twenty local authorities. The new city administration responsible for the whole of Brisbane was established in 1925.

The Brisbane City Council continues to service Australia's largest municipality, with an annual budget of A$1.4 billion. The council is responsible for providing services to 860,000 residents, over 700,000 international and 4.4 million domestic visitors to the city annually, as well as thousands of people who live in adjoining local authority areas and work in the city.

The city of Brisbane covers 1,386 square kilometres (450 square miles), spanning the Brisbane River in a radius up to 25 kilometres from the central business district.

The Brisbane City Council meets community needs for roads, refuse collection, waste recycling, public libraries, botanic gardens, parks, bushland preservation, sporting venues, golf courses, cemeteries, bikeways, swimming pools and community centres. The council also provides water, sewerage and drainage services, as well as buses, ferries and major venues. It regulates property development, building construction, public health standards, environmental standards, city and suburban parking and organises immunisation programmes, community art and free civic concerts.

A call centre, seven customer service centres, five regional business centres, a multimedia kiosk network, an internet site and offices of elected representatives (councillors) provide the customer service interface for these services. The call centre provides telephone services 24 hours a day, 7 days a week and the customer service centres provide face-to-face service delivery throughout Brisbane with operational hours tailored to suit customer requirements. The internet site, with automatic response systems, as of June 2000 was receiving approximately 800 email enquiries per month.

Brisbane City Council operates a sophisticated technology infrastructure and over the past 5 fiscal years has invested A$300 million in technology initiatives in partnership with industry. Brisbane City Council has two large data centres and over 4,700 network connected devices.

In 1994, Brisbane City Council commenced a change journey from a silo-based rules-orientated bureaucracy to an integrated organisation focused around improving services for internal and external customers. The vision of its leaders, the Lord Mayor, Jim Soorley and the Chief Executive Officer, Robert Carter, led to the adoption of a customer service culture that now extends throughout the organisation.

As a result of this process, the council has successfully implemented radical changes in its culture, introduced a clear strategic direction through a corporate planning process, and undertaken management reforms to streamline the organisation and meet competitive testing requirements.

In the decade up to 2000, there have been many changes and milestones for Brisbane City Council resulting from the movement toward an integration of services and systems. The council has focused on its business process and adopted enterprise wide systems to meet its changing business needs.

Some of the major milestones discussed in this case study include:

1994	First corporate plan released to public
1995	Project formed to focus on integrated service delivery
1996	Information resource management architecture delivered
1996	Call centre implemented
1997	Internet and intranet introduced
1998	Separation between corporate functions and specialised operational functions in service delivery and systems
1998	Focus on customer relationship management
1998	Focus on integrated cross-council systems
1998	Mobile office technology introduced
1999	Integrated city assets system introduced
1999	Internet site restructure
1999	Workflow technologies piloted
1999	Year 2000 rectification work
2000	Information resource management architecture revised
2000	Email handling in call centre commenced
2000	E-business and e-commerce activities commenced
2000	Corporate contact system established

Many changes are also occurring in the environment in which the council delivers services. The demographics of Brisbane are changing, there is a separation between the time-rich and time-poor, haves and have-nots, knows and know-nots, social exclusion and inclusion, ethnic diversity and socio-economic levels.

Over the next 12 years, Brisbane is set to become one of the most prosperous cities in the southern hemisphere. Population growth in the Brisbane statistical division averaged 1.9 per cent for the 5 years ending 30 June 1999, the highest of any major city in Australia. In the 12 months to April 2000 employment levels in Brisbane grew by 4 per cent. Brisbane City Council manages this growth and changing city by maintaining a strong community development focus and working closely with the community for the benefit of Brisbane. Brisbane citizens want to be able to influence the decisions and directions of the city, including the types of services and products offered by the council.

The new generation of customers is more technologically aware and competent than ever before. Customers are demanding services to be delivered on-line when they want, where they want and how they want. In contrast, a large proportion of the ageing population is demonstrating preferences for the social contact afforded by face-to-face service.

With technology advancement (internet, digital TV, specialist applications) affording new opportunities in service delivery, the perception of responsiveness to changing customer needs and expectations forms an important element of overall customer satisfaction. In order to continue its record of success Brisbane City Council has had to identify the changes occurring in the customer base and in the environment in which citizens live and work, and respond with products and services that continue to meet the expectations of today and anticipate the demands of the future.

The face of council

In 1995, the council addressed the issue that customers found the organisation difficult to do business with, due to the complex organisational structure and a tendency for work units to operate as independent silos. An integrated customer service project was formed to draw together service delivery across the organisation, focusing initially on counter and telephone services. Council had, at that time, 620 phone numbers listed in the 'White Pages' and provided counter services through seven customer service centres. The project recommended a concept of seamless, anywhere, anytime service delivery through one-stop shop counter and telephone services and a variety of self-help facilities.

It was envisaged that the customer would be able to contact the council via a range of channels including the telephone, mail and the internet from locations including home, libraries and community centres and could access the full range of council services without having to know or understand the organisational structure. This would be achieved through integrated service delivery processes and systems that would provide a consistent window into the council. The systems would direct the customer request to the appropriate department(s) of council and ensure that consistent and accurate responses and feedback were provided to the customer. The structure of these systems is represented in Figures 4.1 and 4.2.

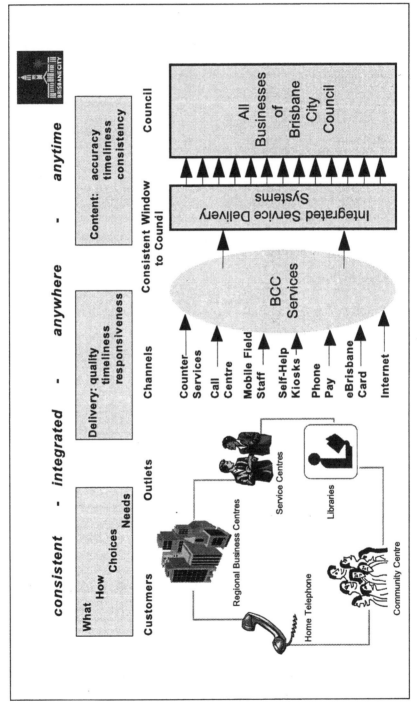

Figure 4.1 Brisbane City Council service delivery platform.

The call centre

The first part of the integrated customer service project involved creating the council's corporate call centre, which was launched in 1996. This centre has developed to the point where it now provides a 7-day 24-hour single contact service for telephone customers.

Two factors were considered critical to the successful implementation of the council's call centre – having the right people in place, and the right processes and systems to support them. To overcome the issues associated with providing front-line response to more than 2,000 services across ten departments of the organisation, the call centre was resourced with highly skilled consultants supported by scripted procedures and answers to ensure the provision of accurate and consistent information and advice.

When the call centre was implemented, the telecommunications systems utilised existing equipment (PABXs, for example) and focused on the require-ments for automated call distribution (ACD), management information systems (ACD/MIS) and rostering/scheduling systems. A major philosophy of the administration was that customers were to speak to a real person, rather than to a machine. Therefore, when you telephone the council, you are connected directly to a consultant and not to interactive voice response (IVR) technology. IVR has always been intended to be used as a support mechanism rather than as the face of council.

Call centre consultants had to be able to access information from a wide variety of operational systems. A comprehensive information repository (knowledge management system) covering the 2,000 council services offered through the channel was a key requirement for the support of service delivery. The Call Centre Information System (CCIS) was built in-house using web technologies, and provided question and answer scripts, pro-cedures, contact details for referrals, access to operational systems and comprehensive searching capabilities.

Every telephone number and customer process incorporated into the call centre was subject to business process re-engineering analysis. The problems experienced by customers were reflected in the multiple iterations experi-enced during the redesign. Many areas considered that their enquiries were too complex to be handled from the call centre and a number of operational areas subsequently struggled to identify irrefutable answers to the inform-ation required in the knowledge system such as:

- What questions do customers ask?
- What are the correct answers?
- Where was this information held?
- Why are customers given different answers on different days and by different people?
- What is the totality of the information the customer needs to know to undertake this function?

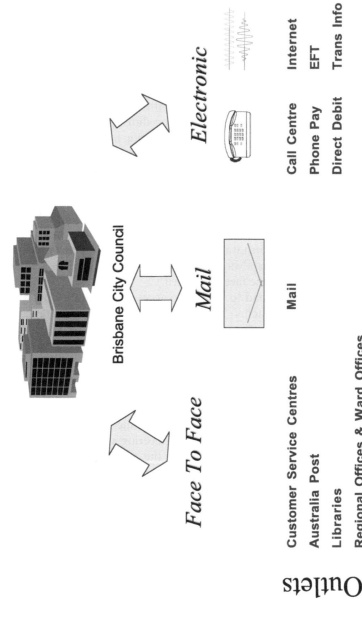

Figure 4.2 Customer channels.

Although council recognised that success in the call centre depended on the effective use of technology, due to the limited time-frame for implementation and the tight budget, a pragmatic approach was taken to the technology systems that support service delivery. Existing technologies and interim solutions were adopted with the expectation that a number of the systems would be replaced within the first years of operation.

The use of web technologies for the call centre information repository was followed in 1997 by the introduction of the council's internet site. Due to the relative infancy of the technologies at that time, content management soon became an issue, with information being duplicated between the systems and having to be maintained separately due to different presentation formats. The complexities contained within undertaking the migration of the council's multimedia kiosk network to web technology exacerbated the issue.

It was always envisaged that the customer service information system would be able to deliver customer contact and service request capabilities to a range of contact channels, not just to the call centre. To achieve this, the system has had to evolve to provide context-sensitive, dynamically generated web pages through:

- Separating content and presentation
- Delivering content and presentation based on identification of the user profile including identity, location, channel and device
- Providing the content owners with the ability to maintain the content without technical tools and professional skills.

The next phase of the integrated service project will deliver a 'desktop' for call centre and customer service centre consultants, with information and screens from existing operational systems seamlessly displayed within the Customer Service Information System (CSIS), which is an extension of the CCIS.

Over 90 per cent of general enquiries received at the call centre are finalised at the first point of contact – this exceeds the council's current corporate key performance indicator. The remaining 10 per cent of calls are referred to specialists from the relevant work units for answering.

To monitor the ongoing effectiveness and efficiency of the call centre, the council has utilised data warehousing tools to provide measures on four key areas – customer service/satisfaction, quality, productivity and staff development. Information in the warehouse comes from a variety of sources including the automated call distributor, performance appraisals, personnel system(s), rework logs, information repository change requests, customer contact system(s) and customer surveys. The warehouse is used to provide management reporting and intelligence and to assist in identifying trends and issues. Current information available through the data warehouse includes average handling time trends for individuals, teams and the call centre, call forecast accuracy and trends, and staffing forecast accuracy.

The call centre is considered world class and was designed for its people, its teams and its customers. It has put the answering of customer enquiries into a team environment with skilled operators, good technology and high service standards. Through the call centre, the council has achieved a common face to the organisation with customer-orientated processes driving the technology. The call centre provides an example of good 'value added' being achieved for customers whilst representing strong cost savings for the council.

Service dynamics

Customer demand for personalised service from organisations is growing. A small business builds relationships with its customers by identifying their needs, remembering their preferences and learning from past interactions how to serve them better in the future. How can the council accomplish something similar when many customers never interact personally with council staff, and where there is customer interaction, it is likely to be with a different employee each time?

The council's services are currently delivered in a generic 'one size fits all' manner. Our knowledge of individual customers is limited, as is our knowledge of our collective customer base. Can the council replicate the creative intuition of the sole proprietor who recognises customers by name, face, and voice and remembers their habits and preferences? In addition, many council businesses are being opened to competition, with some competing externally for work. As a result, the council has corporate customers related to the delivery of services within Brisbane, as well as commercial customers outside the boundaries of Brisbane city.

If the council is to meet the challenge of changing focus from broad market segments to individual customers, we require changes throughout the organisation and information on which to base our strategies. The customer service data warehouse is also being used to collate information regarding customers and contacts across council, to identify trends in customer contacts (by contact type, by customer segment, geographical area for example), to predict customer loyalty and usage, and to identify customer preference patterns.

Systems architecture

As a result of its silo-based history, information technology within the council at the time of the call centre implementation generally comprised work unit-based systems developed in a variety of applications, over a plethora of platforms. These systems were incurring increasingly high costs for maintenance and support. Successful support of the call centre and the many other business changes occurring at that time required council to focus on the information resources and infrastructure required to perform its business functions. In 1996, a high-level information resource management architecture (IRMA) was developed to provide a framework for the planning, management and application of information resources within the council.

IRMA consisted of four dimensions of architecture (work, information, application and technology) which collectively:

- Provided the framework for IT investment decisions based on key services, the consolidation and consistency of information, and the sharing and re-use of application components
- Described a transition strategy for the rationalisation of the diverse systems and applications to enable the migration to a consistent, supportable, manageable technology environment.

The architecture required compliance with important information and technology principles such as:

- Information flows through the organisation must support efficient business processes
- Business processes are to be safeguarded against the impact of failures in any component of their information resources
- Buy not build subject to the overarching principle of cost effectiveness for the council as a whole
- The need to meet evolving business requirements is an important criterion in planning and decisions regarding the acquisition and integration of applications
- Delivery of information should be independent of the delivery channel
- Corporate data, including extensively shared data, should be managed and accessed independent of specific usage functions.

The principles provided a much-needed platform for the organisation to manage its technology effectively and to utilise that technology to support critical business processes. The architecture also addressed a number of business issues emerging from the organisation in response to growing customer expectations and needs. These issues included the dissemination of information via the internet and intranet; support of workgroups and flow of work inefficiencies; flexibility to support change; putting functionality closer to the user and improved delivery mechanisms (including mobile and remote access).

Channel management

One of the issues facing the council in responding to the increased needs and expectations of customers, is to balance the options provided to customers to achieve anywhere, anytime service delivery with the increased costs that those options entail. Evidence both from industry and from within the council indicates that the number of customer contacts is growing annually, yet public entity budgets available to respond to the increased contact volumes remain static (or shrinking).

While it appears on the surface that moving customers to cheaper electronic channels is an easy solution, the public furore experienced by industries who have closed face-to-face channels is an indication that customers have their own views on the issue. Over time customers have developed preferred ways of contacting the council and although these channels may not be the most efficient for the customer or the most cost-effective for the council, as a public service organisation the council has obligations to manage its customers' needs and expectations.

To effectively progress channel migration, it is necessary for the council to not only attract new contacts to lower cost channels, but also to migrate a proportion of existing contacts from higher cost channels to lower cost channels. To achieve this it has been necessary to undertake extensive analysis of existing contacts, identifying who uses which channels, for what services, their motivation in choosing the channel, and the impact of different payment instruments (for example credit cards with frequent flyer programme incentives attached).

Analysis of the total cost of each channel is also required to understand all the cost components of making the channel available to the customer. Channels that appear cost-effective at a first glance often involve a large amount of manual processing and behind the scenes validation, which make the total cost of the channel far higher. The reliance on external channels (agencies) and the impacts of potential closures of those channels must also be factored into any attempt at an accurate costing.

Counter services are by far the council's most costly channel. However customer satisfaction with this channel is also very high. The customer profile shows a definite skew towards the over-forties age group, with payments being the main transaction undertaken. Their preference for this channel relates to the receipt of physical proof of payment. Due to their physical location being within shopping centres, the council's channel services also receive a high percentage of opportunity traffic (drop in trade).

Council's approach to channel management is focused around providing appropriate channel options for products and services. This may result in some products and services offering more channel options than others. A pricing strategy to encourage the use of cost-effective channels and payment instruments is also under consideration. The ultimate outcome is to migrate all easy transactions to electronic channels which progress customer self-help goals, keeping only complex transactions and advice at costly face-to-face channels.

The 'community hub' concept is one approach to maintaining face-to-face contact, while shifting customers to more efficient delivery channels. Community hubs involve co-locating to deliver a synergy of services (virtual and real) that meet the needs of the community. The hubs can also meet the community need for interaction and shared activity, thereby addressing the increased isolation being experienced by some members of our community. Different types of community hubs are being considered in the council including geographic, demographic, recreational and occupational hubs. One of the first examples of the concept is the decision to co-locate customer service centres and libraries. Instead of running two separate facilities in an area, these two customer service functions will be combined in one physical location with integrated services.

In response to the increased usage of the internet as a contact channel, the council has identified the need to transform the existing telephone-based call centre into a multifunctional, multichannel customer contact centre. While initially focusing on the inclusion of responses to email contacts and forms provided on the council's web site, the contact centre could ultimately support many forms of communication including telephone, email, facsimile, interactive chat, escorted browsing and postal mail. This transformation will involve the use of technology such as universal queue management, email response management systems, voice over internet protocol (VOIP), interactive chat, self-help problem resolution, instant messaging and artificial intelligence response systems. Figure 4.3 outlines the structure and functions of the proposed customer contact centre.

The main drivers for the movement to an integrated customer contact centre are the increasing requirements to handle electronic mail received through the council's internet site, and to allocate and track structured electronic forms and applications lodged via the web. The council has been experiencing a large growth in the use of this channel and expects to receive approximately 36,000 emails per month by the year 2001. This estimate is based on the Gartner group's projection that 'by 2001, enterprises will receive more than 25 per cent of their enquiries through the web and internet (0.8 probability)' (Needle 2000: 2).

It is anticipated that the transformation to a customer contact centre will be phased over 4 years. In March 2000, the call centre became the initial point of contact for general email enquiries to the council and also became responsible for monitoring and reporting the council's performance in responding to email. Standard email response templates were developed, and wording and procedures in the customer service information repository were modified to enable call centre staff to cut and paste from the repository into the templates when responding to email enquiries. Automatic acknowledgement was introduced to advise customers of the receipt of their email and email response key performance indicators were agreed for both the call centre and work units.

Approximately 80 per cent of emails received by the council are currently finalised by the call centre at the point of contact, using the existing inform-

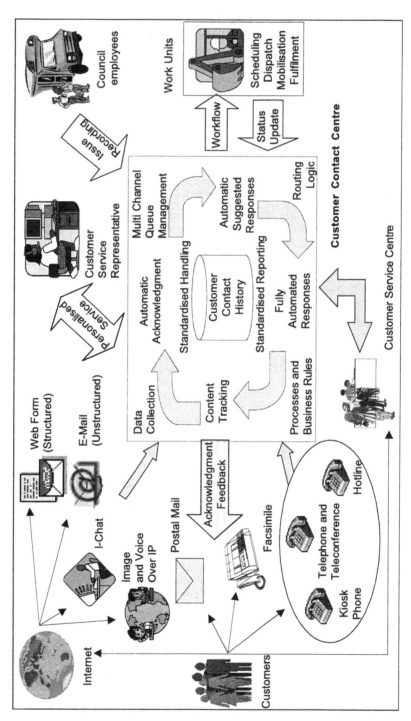

Figure 4.3 Customer contact centre.

ation repository. The remaining 20 per cent are forwarded to work unit specialists for response.

The inclusion of email response in the call centre has resulted in an immediate increase in the level of complexity and diversity handled within this area. Consultants recruited for their telephone skills and customer service focus now require writing skills, email etiquette and internet browsing skills. As the movement to the multimedia contact centre progresses, role requirements include web call-back, web call-through, web chat and escorted browsing. The resultant impact on the call centre is significant, as the average handling time for email response is currently significantly higher than that for telephone handling.

Work units accustomed to responding by letter to postal mail have also experienced skill issues in responding to email. As a result, all email responses are quality assured within the call centre before transmission to customers. Other issues impacting upon service performance include the lack of recognition of email as a legitimate channel, which has resulted in a number of emails forwarded to work units for response being deleted from in-trays or opened and ignored.

Current activities involve the automated logging, tracking and reporting of email, and the logging of email contacts within the council's customer contact system. These activities will have a positive effect on the average handling time for email response and also make the contact history available to other channels, should the customer follow-up their contact via another channel.

Movement to a full email response management system including universal queuing and suggested response systems is not currently considered cost-beneficial, given the council's current email volumes. System design for current activities is, however, designed around the full future solution.

Self-service

The internet is a tool that allows customers to serve themselves, thereby relieving the strain of increased contacts on an organisation. Products and services made available through the internet become as accessible as if the customer made contact through a face-to-face channel. By allowing customers to access information, lodge applications and track the progress of their requests themselves, the council is able to save both valuable customer time and costly employee time.

The council's initial internet site received a large amount of focus, but suffered from a number of design issues including being structured around the council's organisational structure which made it difficult for customers to find content. Following an intensive community consultation process in July 1999, the site was restructured around topics of interest to customers. New content is released to the site every 3 months.

The council's use of the internet goes beyond information delivery and access to the council's services to incorporate a community and lifestyle focus. To reinforce Brisbane as a vital community, the council's internet site aims to provide a service through which communities can gain access to a wide range of information in a manner appropriate to specific community needs. More than 10,000 communities of interest are expected to participate, including individuals with a wide diversity of socio-economic, language and cultural backgrounds, internet experience and interests.

The council's strategy for e-business is to focus on superior service aligned with innovation leading to improved efficiencies over time. The strategy involves:

• Building alliances with partners
• Establishing the council as a trusted leading advisor on community, lifestyle and business
• Creating a portal that is the focal point for interaction between individuals, communities and businesses.

In March 2000, the council released an expression of interest (EOI) to invite responses from interested organisations for creative and innovative solutions, technology, services and products, investment, relationships and business models to contribute to an 'e-Brisbane – Networking Communities and Businesses' initiative. The initiative progresses the vision of Brisbane as a 'smart city' by enabling opportunities for all Brisbane residents, businesses and communities to participate on-line in the new and emerging information economy.

The initiative aims to:

• Promote and maximise access to and the use of on-line services and technology by all Brisbane communities and businesses
• Provide on-line customer-oriented and user-friendly services, which complement existing delivery channels and infrastructure
• Improve the range of packages of information and services available to Brisbane communities and businesses via on-line services
• Contribute to the economic development of Brisbane.

The first deliverable from the EOI will be a portal for Brisbane followed by the introduction of a range of services.

Although much of the focus for the elucidation of an e-business strategy and the development of internet sites and portals is around technology, it has also been necessary for the council to develop policies to ensure effective use and management. Policies identified as critical for the council's portal include brand usage, privacy, security, accessibility, content suitability, external link suitability, copyright, intellectual property, pricing, consumer protection and customer service.

Service delivery is a process

Brisbane city council is committed to becoming the most efficient, effective and customer-oriented public sector administration in Australia. Customer relationship management capabilities are considered critical if the council is to achieve this customer-oriented vision. Efficient and effective customer relationship management requires that Council can register customer contacts, track the status of requests, provide feedback, inform customers on the progress of issues, ensure the satisfactory resolution of customer requests and manage processes using information about resources and key performance indicators.

The call centre and customer service centres provide an effective 'face of council' that meets many of the front-end customer contact needs. However, customer contact is only one step in the end-to-end service delivery process. Successful service delivery involves addressing customers' individual needs and circumstances, keeping customers informed and responding within agreed time-frames.

Research undertaken by the council shows that customers consider that the council's call centre and customer service centres provide polite, courteous, knowledgeable, prompt and reliable services. Their perceptions, however, of the council's fulfilment process (where the work is carried out) are that more focus is required to achieve consistent response times, updates and feedback to the customer and to case manage the completion and closure of requests.

As a result of the council's silo-based past, most of the information technology systems within the council have historically been work unit-based systems incorporating only some of the steps in the service delivery process. The resulting fragmentation of functionality did not ensure that all customer service requests were comprehensively logged, progressed effectively throughout the organisation to the required officers, acted upon within the time specified by council performance standards, or that feedback was provided to the customer regarding progress on the request. The operational systems did not provide any ability to communicate council-wide, support decision-making, or facilitate the ability of work units to work cooperatively in providing a consistent and reliable service experience. In addition, many of the systems supported a decentralised model of customer contact which had all but ended with the introduction of the call centre and customer service centres, and failed to support the new electronic contact opportunities.

In 1998, the council adopted a technology solution concept to address the requirements of both a corporate view and a business view of systems delivery. It was agreed that a number of steps in the service delivery process would be delivered through corporate solutions (customer contact, allocation, payment, status tracking, dispatch, mobilisation, feedback, closure), while other steps in the process could be delivered through operational systems (for example, application assessment, scheduling, fulfilment, compliance checking). End-to-end service delivery would be achieved through the use of a series of corporate and specialist operational applications, achieving both corporate management requirements and local business requirements (Figure 4.4).

It was agreed that customer requests and complaints would be captured at the point of contact (counter, telephone, mail, fax, internet, multimedia) and tracked by other systems through job allocation, scheduling, dispatch, mobilisation, fulfilment by operational staff, and closure. The systems would ensure the customer was provided with feedback at all relevant points in the process and that the service status would be shared amongst stakeholders.

The proposed corporate customer contact functionality required each customer contact to be logged and associated with other contacts relating to the same matter. Ultimately the complete case history of the progress on a customer request/complaint would be updated from other systems and made available to contact channels through this single system for customer feedback and follow-up. This approach would ensure that all duplicate service requests were identified at the point of contact and would eliminate omissions or conflicting information being held in multiple systems. The implementation of a corporate system would only be the first step, however, as customer contact functionality was scattered throughout multiple operational systems. Interfaces mimicking the contact functionality had to be developed to ensure that the systems continued to function. Ultimately, contact functionality will be stripped from each of the legacy systems and interfaces will be developed to provide the source information for processing.

Following the architecture's 'buy not build' principle, an extensive tendering process was undertaken with numerous customer relationship management (CRM) solutions meeting the required customer contact functionality. In each case, however, the solution was not feasible due to the licence fees incurred in making the contact logging functionality available to all 6,000 council staff, the system integration required to fit to the council's architecture and the requirement to integrate with existing systems. Accordingly, the council resorted to an in-house development option based on its new Java/CORBA/middleware environment.

The new corporate and business systems delivery system was implemented in August 2000. It not only fundamentally changed the way the call centre and customer service centres processed contacts, but also represented the council's first foray into object-oriented technologies. As a corporate customer contact tool, generic functionality useable across the whole organisation was required rather than tailoring the functionality specifically to the initial channels. Managing the expectations of users accustomed to being provided with tailored solutions was possibly the biggest challenge in system development and implementation.

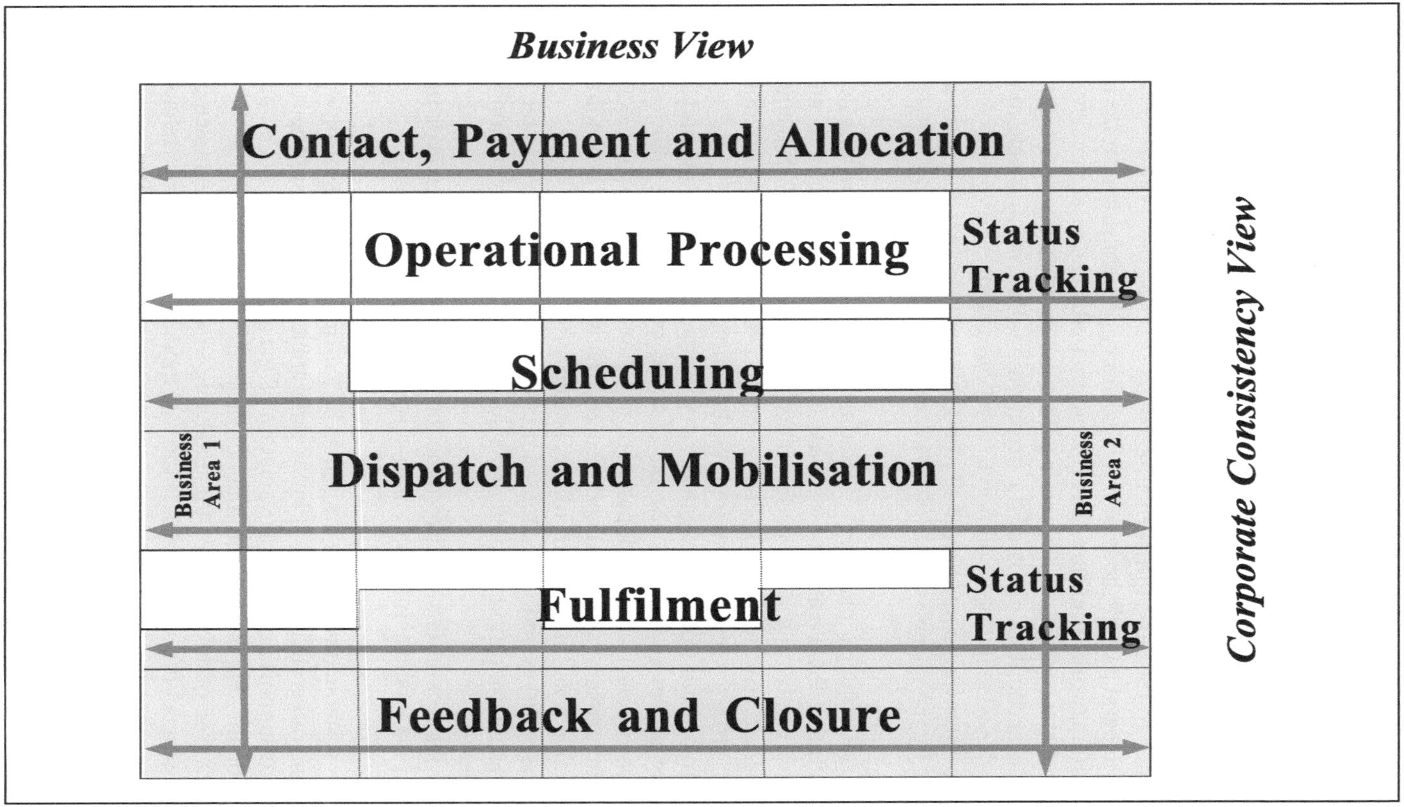

Figure 4.4 Service delivery model.

The back room

Although much of the technology application in the council is focused on the highly visible front end, technologies are also being widely utilised to support work units involved in end-to-end service delivery.

Brisbane City Council's infrastructure assets are valued in excess of A$15 billion. The City Assets System introduced in July 1999 has developed from the need to realise the inherent benefits from a total asset management approach to the city's infrastructure assets.

An integral part of the system is the delivery of a consistent works management framework to ensure that operational efficiencies are achieved in all areas of the council. By combining the total asset management philosophy with the accounting needs of the organisation, the system is able to offer an enterprise-wide business solution to asset ownership.

The following components of the asset management life cycle are supported by the system:

- Asset strategic planning – including the high-level functions needed to optimise the life and use of assets over their full life cycle (i.e. modelling and forecasting asset performance, budgeting, risk management and management reporting). The system provides the necessary information for strategic replacement and rehabilitation decisions.
- Project and works management – covering all the planning and scheduling processes required for the creation of assets, the maintenance of existing assets and the donation of new assets from third-party developers. Management of capital and recurrent budgets through expenditure programs is an integral part of this business function.
- Asset survey and inspection – for condition assessment, and the ranking and identification of potential maintenance and rehabilitation requirements.
- Asset accounting – to determine the value of assets, depreciate them and report financial information to corporate financial systems.

The system consolidates a number of existing asset maintenance systems into one integrated system. It holds geographical location, sufficient information to support an auditable valuation of the assets and works management functionality for the programming of projects.

A 'whole of life' concept for managing assets has been implemented to optimise asset life and introduces forecast modelling to enhance rehabilitation decisions. A set of corporate consistencies related to strategies, processes and standards for asset management was included in the change management activities required to support the system. The council's corporate asset knowledge base is now shared to support the council initiatives, such as the call centre.

The asset system will deliver substantial and on-going benefits to the council, including a reduction in the base level of the planned maintenance budget and a reduction of resource consumption in the order of 5 to 10 per cent of the infrastructure rehabilitation budget.

The asset system will be responsible for managing information about both financial and non-financial asset classes. Financial asset classes are those assets for which financial information will appear in the council's books of account. The classes of financial assets that will be supported are set out in Table 4.1.

In addition to financial assets, the system manages information about assets for which financial information is not reported in the council's books of account, as shown at Table 4. 2.

In 1998, the council introduced computing technologies into vehicles, enabling Council officers to function in 'mobile offices'. This initiative allows officers to receive and accept tasks assigned to them, print standard letters, and interrogate case histories and local information. Increased time in the field has resulted in productivity improvements of up to 1 day per week per officer. Other mobile solutions have followed, including the use of palm technologies which download asset information, update asset conditions in the field and upload work orders on their return to the office.

Table 4.1 Brisbane City Council span of responsibility 1

Bikeways	Lined/Unlined engineered drainage systems
Bridges	Major traffic directional signs
Buildings	parks assets
Buses and Ferries	Retaining walls
City fleet assets	Road pavement
Culverts	Sea walls, river walls and groynes
Enclosed stormwater drainage network	Surfaced medians
Fences	Traffic signal network
Flood mitigation schemes	Water and sewerage assets
Footpaths	Wharves, piers and jetties
Kerb and channel network	Council land

Table 4.2 Brisbane City Council span of responsibility 2

Bus shelter sheds	Natural waterways and creeks
Grass cutting areas	Parking meters
Landscaped areas	Parking signs
Landscaping	Parks assets parking signs
Line marking	Plans and designs
Litter bins	Seats
Natural environment assets	Traffic signs

While the use of mobile offices and mobile technologies in the council has delivered productivity improvements, their introduction has raised a range of issues including:

- Bandwidth required to deliver database interrogation capabilities
- Coverage of telco communications network
- Culture change required in work areas used to working from an office
- The expense of the equipment required
- Organisational infrastructure requirements
- Occupational health and safety issues
- Thin client applications
- Rapidly changing technologies in the network transmission field.

Occupational health and safety issues addressed in the use of mobile office technologies included:

- The requirement to twist and lean to use the keyboard, screen and printer
- Glare problems due to exposure to sunlight
- Eye strain due to small screen characters
- Typing difficulty due to key size.

The requirement for mobile office technology varies greatly between work units. Some areas merely need the capability to deliver work requests while others need full task acceptance capabilities and data base interrogation. The council is currently developing a panel of technology options for mobile office solutions.

It is envisaged that a workflow technology will be used in the process management to transfer work electronically between the steps in the service delivery process, time-keep the progress within each step and within the total process, to escalate service failures and to provide work volume reports.

During 1999/2000 process mapping was undertaken on all processes within one branch of the council. Three service delivery processes were re-engineered and workflowed. Key issues emerging from the pilot study included:

- Recognising that many benefits are achieved through process re-engineering and this step should be considered mandatory (up to 20 per cent efficiency savings).
- The benefits of workflow in managing the delivery process can be achieved without the need to manage activities at a low level.
- The use of consultants to undertake re-engineering activities is not sustainable.
- Not all processes will benefit from the use of workflow technology.
- Many service delivery processes fit the same generic workflow process.

- Integration between workflow, document management and imaging technologies provided some additional productivity savings in work units where correspondence is a critical part of the process.

Following on from the success of the workflow pilot, the council saw the acquisition of the workflow, document management and imaging software as the provision of core corporate infrastructure. Since the tools were to be used to provide functionality across a number of projects, a corporately consistent technology solution was considered. However, investigations within the council indicated that while the functional and technical requirements for workflow were consistent across the council, they varied considerably for document management and imaging.

The council has not yet been successful in procuring an affordable off-the-shelf integrated solution for workflow, document management and imaging technologies to support end-to-end management of service delivery processes. Fit with architecture, lack of integration between components, user and server licensing costs, and lack of local support and expertise feature highly in the issues addressed to date.

Year 2000

Undertaking year 2000 rectification work afforded the opportunity to review every system in the council and evaluate whether the system should:

- continue to be used
- be replaced with updated technology
- be retired
- be incorporated into other systems.

The process proved useful to the council. Many systems were retired outright and others were amalgamated with systems of like functionality.

Seamless government

At a time when customers are expecting to receive higher levels of service and reductions in the cost of government, customers do not distinguish between local authority boundaries or between the services provided by different levels of government. When dealing with government, customers want services delivered quickly and efficiently regardless of the agency providing the service.

Seamless government is an emerging strategic theme in twenty first century governance aimed at achieving integrated customer service outcomes through horizontal (across local authorities) and vertical (between levels of government) alignment of public sector administrations. The model delivers services from the point of view of the customer who prefers to have an event or situation taken care of by one, or at most a few, service provider(s). Such seamlessness can enable integrated billing and payment, single notification of change of address, and the processing of the outcomes of life events such as births, deaths and marriages. Seamlessness can also enable private sector utilities and public sector corporations to address issues such as integrated meter reading and utility billing.

Seamless government can only be achieved through the use of cross-functional teams and often cross-organisational teams, shifting from a focus on internal activities to a design focused on customer outcomes. The goal is to shed bureaucratic control and compliance, reconfigure the segmented pieces around lean streamlined principles, and organise governance in an holistic manner.

Information technology is creating important opportunities and methods for governments to work together to improve and deliver services. It is also revolutionising the seamless delivery of services to customers by speeding up internal operations, providing easier access to services and integrating information across the public sector. In Brisbane, information regarding neighbouring local authorities, state and federal government has been included in the call centre information repository since its introduction in 1996.

The challenge for Brisbane City Council is to work together with other governments using both a horizontal (across local authorities) and vertical (across tiers of government – federal, state, local) approach to provide integrated seamless services. This will involve joint planning, integration of programs and better use of both social and technological infrastructure. It will also require removing regulatory duplication and inconsistency in standards and policies.

Conclusion

Many public administrations, including Brisbane city council, have historic-ally assumed more and more responsibilities and assigned the administration and operation of their functions to functionally delineated sections of the administration. This council has worked to change the values and culture of the organisation through emphasising customer first, fairness and equity, respect for people, quality, and communication. With the theme of customer service as the light on the hill, walls affecting service delivery have been dissolved and flexible customer oriented processes and systems have been designed. Brisbane city council has become a virtual organisation with many partnerships and networks blurring the boundaries of the organisation.

Council has been a major user of technology to support changes and efficiencies occurring in the organisation. At times the complexity and sheer volume of technology projects under way has created problematic issues.

Multiple information technology projects focused on a particular operational area can cause organisational stress and service reduction due to the number of operational staff required for user representation, design, testing and training.

Due to the council's size and the range of services provided, the procurement of standardised local government application software has proven to be a challenge. The regionalised approach to service delivery and the number of users involved in operational activities often challenges the design and architecture of 'off-the-shelf' software. The concept of buying a package to meet business requirements has also proven difficult in environments where the process is driven by legislation and adaptation to fit the technology is therefore not possible.

The council's information technology architecture has delivered improvements over the council's previously fragmented systems development approach. The architecture has limited the number of application types and hardware platforms requiring support which has halted the ever-increasing costs of maintaining the council's environment. The ability of software vendors to meet the council's architectural requirements does, however, continue to be an issue.

Current focus within the council is on achieving still greater levels of value for money expenditure in information technology and focusing on whether the council is developing luxury systems with custom features or pragmatic fit-for-purpose functionality. Whilst legislative and critical functionality are considered mandatory, a balance between optional functionality and the provision of features and usability is being addressed in system approvals and design. In areas such as customer services where staff are required to access many operational systems, the integration of those systems on to the desktop and the creation of interfaces between systems which share data have proved challenging.

Real improvements in the council's customer satisfaction and service performance have resulted from the movement to an integrated approach to both service delivery and systems development. Through its size and focus Brisbane city council has the capacity to truly deliver integrated services to its citizens.

References

Australia (1924) *City of Brisbane Act,* Brisbane: GOPRINT.
Needle, P. (2000) *Customer Relationship Management: Using IT to Put Focus on the Customer – Report No. 5701,* Connecticut: Gartner Direct Products.

Chapter 5

Beyond 20/20 vision, improving the human condition

A Canadian perspective

Dawn Nicholson-O'Brien

Knowledge and creativity are the drivers in this economy.

(Cappe 2000a)

As we believe, so shall we lead

Governments exist, ultimately, to improve human well-being. When our descendants write the history of our times, from the perspective of a few hundred years, they may well record an unprecedented change in the human condition. For the first time in human history, more people in the world are literate and can read and write than those who can not (Massé 2000). Thus, ever growing numbers of people have choices to exercise as never before in the history of mankind. Canadian citizens, and the civil servants who serve them, are seeking new 'return on investment' opportunities. Governments are learning to be trendsetters, not followers, in order to anticipate and surpass citizen expectations.

Our new 'mental geography' globally is serving to shift traditional analytical thinking from a framework that asks 'what is governance?' to an act of inquiry, specifically, 'what can governance be?' Within this context, governments can no longer cling to a simple economic productivity model, which focuses primarily upon minimising risks, maximising efficiencies, and creating stability. Innovation and creativity are the 'rocket fuel' of the knowledge-based economy.

Knowledge workers, who deal with exceptions and the unknown daily, are designing a desired future that supports all citizens in attaining their human potential. In the midst of global discussions regarding the burgeoning bioeconomy, complexity science and the wonders of modern technology, Canada is asking 'what do we need to preserve that makes us uniquely human?' and 'what can we do to create a better future?'

The Clerk of Canada's Privy Council, Mel Cappe, in addressing over 600 federal executives, observed that while Bill Gates can correctly refer to 'business @ the speed of thought', good government must occur 'at the speed of the public interest' (Cappe 2000b). In his speech, Cappe described the current breed of civil servant as 'fonctionnaires sans frontières', encouraging us as public servants to design permeable borders instead of strong walls, thereby gestating the seeds of learning for the new millennium.

Living in an era of extraordinary possibilities

Stability and the safety of organisational 'boxology' have all but disappeared in the knowledge-based economy we now call home. We are embracing very deliberately a degree of chaos, in the absence of which there can be no innovation. As Bourgon (1999) suggests, 'There's order in madness'. Jocelyne Bourgon, the President of Canada's Centre for Management Development (CCMD), and Canada's former Clerk of the Privy Council, has been at the forefront of developing and leading change in the Canadian federal context. She shepherded the Canadian federal government through what was arguably one of the most challenging periods of its 233-year existence.

During the 7-year period ending in 1999, the Government of Canada emerged from a dramatic period of necessary debt and deficit reduction to help restore the country to economic health. The Prime Minister of Canada, the Right Honourable Jean Chrétien, sums up the achievements of this period:

> In just 7 years, Canada has gone from the worst recession since the 1930s to the longest economic expansion since the 1960s. From being called a candidate for the Third World by the Wall Street Journal to what the London Financial Times now calls the second miracle economy in North America . . . our books are balanced. We are paying down our public debt. The provinces have done the same. . . . We are among the G-7 leaders in economic growth and job creation. Our productivity tripled last year. Indeed, we are on a run of economic growth that has never before been recorded in Canada . . . and to get Canadians ready to prosper in the knowledge-based economy . . . and Canada continues to set the international standard for quality of life. For the last 6 years in a row, the United Nations has rated Canada as the best place in the world in which to live.
>
> (Chrétien 2000)

A springboard for renewal

The model used to achieve program review tests for this period of downsizing was uniquely Canadian. Jocelyne Bourgon observes, 'when you reach a plateau, you must use it as a springboard'.

While governments all over the world were focusing on how to do more with less, during this economic downturn, the Canadian federal government chose to tackle economic restraint, reengineering and restructuring. Key to this review in Canada, referred to as 'Getting Government Right', was a series of public interest tests that were applied. This resulted in a recommitment to Canadian and public service values, an enhanced focus on results, putting the citizen first, and new reporting, transparency and accountability measures.

Half a dozen strategic initiatives launched during this 7-year period are now yielding fruit and hold the keys to the rebirth of the public service (PS) of Canada. The magic of the Canadian reform, Jocelyne notes, was the synergy between initiatives, not simply a clarity of purpose married with efficiency. This intricate 'spider's web' led to the creation of a futures-oriented public policy research network with roots in all parts of society. The Task Force on Public Service Values and Ethics, led by John Tait, was the bedrock, foundation and anchor for these other measures. In this ground-breaking report, Tait and his co-contributors noted: 'we do not learn about the (public) good from abstractions but rather from encountering it in real life, in the flesh and blood of a real community and real people' (Tait 1996, reprinted with dedication, January 2000).

Leadership in the knowledge-based economy

We are articulating what the role of a leader is in the knowledge-based economy. Of course, globally, there are examples of countries that have embarked upon the creation of their own learning societies. In a world with neither friends nor enemies, only competitors, the challenge will be to benchmark our progress against that of other countries (Conference Board of Canada 2000). Are we up to the challenges of serving citizens in a connected society and in a connected world? Citizens will ultimately be the judge.

This is a journey of 'what has the power to be', Bourgon argues (Bourgon 2000). It is, at its heart, a journey from the machine model of the industrial era, to a human ecology, from the death of the 'organisation man or woman' to the birth of knowledge entrepreneurs who belong to many 'tribes', but to no one organisation and who are passionate iconoclasts. It is a journey from a unicentric governance model to one that is polycentric, from an economy that exploits physical capital and financial wealth, to one where ideas, applied knowledge and innovation are the new currency.

If we, in Canada, are not at the leadership 'edge', then we need to be. The market is free to bear selected parts of the leadership responsibility. In governments, we need to work with all of our citizens, sectors, political and democratic institutions, to serve our society well in an era of connectedness. The final test will be how relevant we are to the society that we serve.

The 'midwives' of a new Canadian public service

In this chapter you will be introduced to some of the pioneers who are transforming Canada's PS and Canadian society. Many of these pioneers are creating powerful human communities of practice or communities of interest that make organisational, sectoral or geographic boundaries meaningless. For the purposes of this chapter, nearly thirty such leaders were interviewed.

The *Oxford English Dictionary* defines the word 'ordinary' as meaning 'regular, normal, customary, usual, not exceptional, not above the usual, common place'. However, in 20 years of public service I have never met anyone remotely resembling an 'ordinary citizen', nor have I met an 'average public servant'. The citizens we serve are extraordinary human beings and our political masters and public servants are no less so. The leaders discussed here are serving as catalysts for personal awakening in their organisations and as catalysts for wider societal renewal. They have chosen to serve as unofficial midwives for the creation of a new public service.

Failure is not an option

Keith Coulter, of the Treasury Board Secretariat of Canada (TBS), suggests that as with the launch of the Apollo 13 and man's journey to the surface of the moon, 'failure is not an option' in implementing a modern management framework for the PS of Canada. *Results for Canadians*, this framework, is helping us to identify what constitutes a world-class performance in each part of our operating universe. Within this context, a 'four points commitments compass' has been constructed, revolving around four key management commitments; a citizen focus, a clear set of values guiding management decisions, the achievement of results and responsible spending (Treasury Board Secretariat of Canada 2000).

Importantly, in an era when we are beginning to make new strategic investments in our society (Martin 2000a, b), there is a need to have a better understanding of federal performance and results – results that are directly relevant to policy discussions. Mike Joyce, the TBS assistant secretary responsible for expenditure management and strategic planning, notes that this new management framework we have developed will permit us to subtract some of our former responsibilities to make way for new innovative roles. The planned abandonment of what no longer serves us well and adaptability are seen as being keys to success.

The 'F' words

Where governments have succeeded in helping create huge breakthroughs in medical science, in international trade, in human global security or in new governance agreements for social union, it is usually because we have overcome the fear of failure. This is not always easy to do since governments are subject to constant public and media scrutiny and risk-taking is more complex in this environment.

In traditional government organisations, people with innovative ideas must submit their ideas to established institutional guardians in order to secure funding for their programme or service. In knowledge-based organisations federally, quite the reverse is true, as leaders vie to attract the best new ideas and regard 'failure' as a high value learning opportunity. So stewardship, then, while important, must also leave room for innovation and for unorthodox thinking.

Dr Alexander Himelfarb, Deputy Minister for Canadian Heritage (Canadian Heritage 2000), argued that he wanted to insert another 'F' word into the dialogue around what is required to create high-functioning knowledge-based workplaces – the word 'fun'. He reasoned that human beings are, by definition, creative when they feel most joyful and most secure in relationships of trust. However, the history of most public institutions, other than in times of great crisis, has often been about rewarding leaders for 'playing it safe'. The key test in this era should be 'what has this leader done for Canada?' and 'how have they developed other human beings to liberate their full potential?'

The anatomy of human progress

Never in the history of the human race has the past been a worse guide to the creation of our future. For newly cyber-literate children, and for the Nexus generation, business and creativity have much in common with play. Our next-generation leaders can pick and choose their employer, dictating the terms of their talent offering. Within this context, there are no false choices between a life of contemplation or a life of commerce, between a life spent pursuing the public good or financial success, or between healthy and 'anorexic' organisations.

Himelfarb describes a world where we are undergoing what he terms a 'species change'. The Greek businessman wearing a toga in the ancient Athens agora, the Venetian or Roman merchant in Italy in the fifteenth century, the Victorian industrialist in the nineteenth century, and the venture capitalists of today are dramatically different 'species' he argues. Change is occurring so quickly in our world that we are living it as a cyber-revolution, in real-time, not as a historical analysis or retrospective that permits reflection. The dynamic social and human context within which knowledge is created today is extremely fluid.

The original automakers or inventors of 'horseless carriages', the early pioneers of flight and aviation, the doctors advancing the notion of bacteria, or the first astronomers, all had to generate knowledge of something that could exist yet did not exist. These very leaps of ingenuity represent the anatomy of human progress.

Life sciences and Canada's Institutes for Health Research (CIHR)

In the Canadian context, every great federal breakthrough has been accomplished through what we might refer to as experimental groups or innovation-based communities. The new Canadian Institutes of Health Research is, accordingly, a hybrid organisation of the best kind. A national task force on health research (Health Canada 2000), made up of representatives from across the entire health research community in Canada, reported in 1998 that there was an exciting opportunity to develop a comprehensive and interactive approach to health research. Guided by these recommendations the federal government announced the creation of the Canadian Institutes of Health Research (CIHR) in its 1999 budget. Distinguished scientists, leading academics, educators, health practitioners, social scientists, along with representatives of the voluntary and private sectors came together to provide advice on legislation and on the governance of CIHR (House of Commons 2000).

The CIHR was officially launched on 7 June, 2000 (CIHR 2000). An innovative agency, it is responsible for funding health research in Canada and the creation of new health knowledge, intended to be translated into improved health for Canadians, more effective health services and products and a strengthened health care system. It was organised through a framework of thirteen 'virtual' institutes, each dedicated to a specific area of focus, bringing together researchers pursuing common goals. The four pillars of the CIHR include biomedical, clinical science, health systems and services, and the social, cultural and other factors that affect the health of populations. These institutes represent powerful human communities of practice and of interest.

To ensure talented investigators are provided with the resources and training needed to address the health challenges faced by Canadians, the CIHR's budget is posited to be $402 million in 2000–2001, rising to $533 million in following fiscal years. This is intended to allow Canada to keep its best and brightest scientists and remain internationally competitive in today's knowledge-based economy. The resulting benefits to Canadians include both health and economic dividends, along with powerful knowledge-generating partnerships helping to articulate the public interests inherent in health research. The research will remain in the public domain. Importantly, members of Parliament and senators were extremely active and supportive in bringing the CIHR to life.

Karen Mosher, the Executive Director of the CIHR referred to the newly created entity as 'the ultimate expression of connected leadership – leadership that we are seeing from all of the interrelated human networks'. The Institutes are very deliberate community hubs with spokes radiating outwards to ensure that our high-value health knowledge is captured and shared for the benefit of Canadians.

Importantly, Mosher referred specifically to the challenges of marrying the scientific, public policy and values issues juxtaposed in the bioeconomy, commenting, 'ready or not, it's a phenomenon like globalisation hitting us and the CIHR will help to construct informed public debate, not just a knee-jerk reaction'.

Leadership in action at the National Judicial Institute

George Thomson, the executive director of Canada's National Judicial Institute, is at the heart of a rich knowledge network linking federally appointed judges in the highest courts of the land. Out of 1,000 federal judges, 700 judges have made a commitment to on-line learning and knowledge transfer that includes everything from electronic benchbooks to being able to go on-line with another judge in a real-time courtroom hearing. E-learning and what might be termed 'e-literacy' for Canada's judges supplements annual conferences and forums where judges come together to learn about the latest developments shaping the justice system. In June 2000, for example, hundreds of Canada's top judges met in Kananaskis, Alberta, to discuss with medical and other experts some of the legal, ethical and public policy challenges inherent in converging biomedical, medical–legal and technological issues.

This brave new world being navigated by Canada's judges is far from being the only test of their leadership and evolving knowledge. Canada's judges, the National Judicial Institute, and partners are joining forces to provide international judicial education around the globe. Countries from Russia to Nepal have sought Canada's assistance in reinventing their courts and justice systems, complete with just-in-time judicial education and on-line, multi-media judicial networks.

In this context of continuous learning and knowledge capture Canada's Chief Justice of the Supreme Court of Canada, the Honourable Justice Beverley McLachlin (Tibbetts 2000), noted that one of her top goals is to improve judges' education and knowledge so they are prepared to deal with new issues in society. To support this a 'futures committee' has been established to track emerging legal trends and problems. The National Judicial Institute provides a structure to ensure that Canada is at the leading edge, globally, of judicial education and review processes.

Challenging organisational 'surrogates'

Peter DiGiammarino, the CEO of Intelliven, a corporation located in the USA, speaks eloquently of the complexity facing governments, and corporations in this emerging knowledge economy. He points out that part of the discomfort governments and corporations are experiencing in this millennium is that as organisations designed to sustain themselves, they are being asked to replace themselves and to reinvent what remains.

He notes that Charles Rossotti, the head of the American Internal Revenue Service, assumed this role with the IRS after coming from a private sector executive role with American Management Systems (AMS). Case studies and reports, Charles Rossotti quickly learned, became surrogate experiences for actually fast-tracking modern governance reforms. Rossotti's response was to take members of Congress and other opinion leaders on a bus tour to visit institutions where clients were being treated in a very different way. As a result of this awareness-raising exercise, he subsequently received approval for making the significant changes that he identified as being necessary to ensure an improved tax system.

The challenge in an established organisation, where one variable has been optimised and drives business planning, is recognising that there are multiple variables driving our lives now.

Rossotti's experience is surely evidence that establishing a basis for moving forward in an organisational context must involve challenging accepted models of practice and mindsets. This is further evidence of the fact that knowledge is constantly evolving and that human identity evolves with it.

An important learning agenda

John Manley, Canadian Minister of Foreign Affairs and International Trade, and formerly Canada's industry minister, is a leader with an exciting story to tell about Canada seizing the connectivity agenda more rapidly than any other country. He is, for example, proud that the establishment of Canada's SchoolNet is said to predate the incorporation of even Netscape. Minister Manley notes that the Canadian government was one of the few countries to see the potential for digital inclusion of citizens on our cyberways as a social issue, intrinsic to being a learning society. Manley observes that what has set Canada apart from others around the world is our ability to 'see innovation as a system'. By building on human networks in our society, by creating centres of excellence, we have been able to conduct leading-edge research on networking concepts.

As the only non-European member of the European Space Agency and in other international scientific bodies, Canada has strong scientific expertise and receives significant returns from our related investments in human knowledge networks.

Partnerships around genomics and proteomics are but one example of the importance of the cross-pollination of ideas and of people. Our very openness to ideas is a net gain for Canada, especially in an era of curiosity-driven research.

Minister Manley predicts that, in 3 years' time, Canada will be in a position to share even more of our specialised knowledge. The country has the 'learnware' or the capacity to share advanced multi-media applications in the healthcare field, for example. He notes the need to distinguish our specialised knowledge found in Montreal, Toronto and elsewhere from that of other cities like Boston or Chicago.

On 16 October, 2000, Minister Manley announced the creation of a national broadband task force to advise the Government of Canada on how best to make high-speed broadband internet services available to citizens and businesses in Canada by 2004. He emphasises:

> If we are really saying that we will bring the Canadian content that is respectful of knowledge and that is info-driven, the technological platform has to be there to create the super-structure we want to create Canadian economic opportunities and to preserve our values.

Within this opportunity-driven vision, Manley depicts a fascinating kaleidoscope of the human family. Time, space and distance, he notes, have essentially been rendered irrelevant by a collection of modern technologies. He viewed the Olympics in Sydney, Australia, in real-time from the comfort of his own home. He watched the Iron Curtain and the Berlin Wall crumble under the unrelenting eye of the world media.

The breakdown of tribalism and nationalism offers, he suggests, the opportunity for much greater commonality in the human family, enabling poorer countries to share in global prosperity increasingly, while also highlighting a gap that has been exacerbated between knowledge-rich and knowledge-poor countries.

This extended period of prosperity and growth, he believes, is 'scooping up' people in our society who have often been left out of the workforce. His own measure of a truly inclusive and great society is one that reaches out to all citizens to ensure that each person can embrace and experience this prosperity.

He notes the progress that he and his government have made in addressing early childhood development issues, creating the basic building blocks for healthy economic and social participation in our society. Those who are disadvantaged are the very people we need to support in our knowledge-rich society.

Improving the human condition is never far from his mind. He cites the 'mind-boggling work' being undertaken by some of his civil servants – one in particular, Mary Frances Laughton, who is the Chief of the Assistive Devices Industry Office. He calls her a 'guardian angel'. Laughton and group help people who are blind or disabled to participate in our society via the development of assistive devices. Our digital world, he observes, has allowed extraordinary people like Stephen Hawking to shine through – a wheelchair-bound astronomer and physicist whose groundbreaking work is world-class. He wants Canada's citizens to be able to light up our society with their ideas and spirit.

A quest for meaning

Christine Nymark, a newly appointed Assistant Deputy Minister, and former Director General of Life Sciences with Industry Canada, talks about the significant reinvestment in science federally during the last few years to support what is termed 'serious discovery research'. She was instrumental, in 2000, in creating Genome Canada.

In the quest for breakthrough knowledge and improved human well-being, she notes that we cannot rest on our achievements and describes the need for additional flexibility to ensure improved federal partnerships in discovery research. She articulates a view that young people, with academic excellence, need more financial freedom to be able to pursue breakthrough research in high-value knowledge domains. However, while acknowledging that there have been key investments federally and provincially in science and technology research, she emphasises the need to invest more in humanities research, what she calls 'the other half of the knowledge picture'. As we come forward with extraordinary scientific and technological discoveries that can change people's lives, Christine Nymark believes that we need to understand the values system underpinning the use of these discoveries. In particular, educating public servants to think about the future in a very different way, where they do not simply extrapolate from what they already know, to project a future, but rather create a better future, is part of the role she sees for key senior public service managers.

Nymark advocates the benefits of having a knowledgeable workforce that is far more mobile, where people come into the federal government for a few highly beneficial years and then move into other parts of society, weaving a vital knowledge web as they do so. Additionally, she places a high premium on creative policy thinking. She wants thinkers to be seen as essential investments in our future, not as crude overheads. The best teams, in her view, like society more generally, benefit from a clear identity, solid values and an inclusive character. Such an approach should stimulate creativity and foster trust in the workplace, providing for the emergence and nurturing of a culture where 'doing good' is achieved organically.

Everybody in

Canada's innovative use of the internet, of modern satellite, telecommunications and wireless technologies is the direct result of fostering symbiotic partnerships between the voluntary sector, public and private sectors.

In the 'Connecting Canadians' strategy, originally devised by Industry Canada with many private sector, educational and other partners, the guiding principle has been one of 'digital inclusion', rather than that of 'digital divide'. Canadians now enjoy among the highest penetration of home computers and the widest access to cable systems in the world. Canada also has the most advanced fibre-optic network in the world and was similarly a pioneer in connecting all schools and libraries to the internet. As Doug Hull, Industry Canada's Director General of the Information Highways Applications branch comments, given its geographic size, Canada could not have been developed without the creative use of technological and other partnerships.

In the internet field, Canada's SchoolNet, digital collections and community access programmes (Industry Canada 1999a), have resulted from partnerships between governments, business and the non-profit sector working together to ensure internet access for Canadians long before the marketplace would normally make it available.

By contrast, he describes the American approach to making technology accessible to citizens as a 'trickle-down approach'. Canada, on the other hand has chosen a model of 'everybody in'.

By connecting the young minds of tomorrow in schools and by reaching children in the far north of Canada's Nunavut, programmes such as SchoolNet (Industry Canada 1999b) create universal public access to information, and provide the social web of belonging that draws us together. Access points include schools, public libraries and even lighthouses. Communities and schools select their own sites.

On this subject, Hull again reflecting on the Canadian/USA examples of practice, puts forward a view that in the USA, with a population of approximately 260 million people, the federal government has introduced 1,000 public internet access sites to date. Hull compares this with Canada's investment in up to 10,000 sites of public access to serve a population of only 30 million people.

However, the more important question, he suggests, is to focus upon what people are doing with the connectivity they enjoy and when they are engaged, how this creates a stronger economy and culture, not just a better government service offering. The 'citizen to community to country' aspect, as Hull terms it, is helping to move Canada along a development and knowledge spectrum, along with countries like Sweden and Finland. The internet is a powerful tool for disseminating community-based economic and social development techniques and opportunities.

It was this kind of understanding of the potential of the 'tool' that was behind the creation of Canada's SchoolNet program. SchoolNet won the 1998 International Innovation Award of the Commonwealth Association for Public Administration and Management and had to achieve a consensus across levels of government in order to deliver results optimally. There was an agreement on the part of provincial and federal governments to lay aside competing agendas in favour of a unifying common purpose to install information technology and internet access and to train teachers in order to accelerate the learning rates of children. From the standpoint of developing rich human networks, cooperation between governments, industry, educators and children has not only created more feedback loops for innovation, but also a willingness to build 'another big innovation'.

Hull notes that the same model underlines the community access programme which is providing universal public internet access for all Canadians through 10,000 public access sites. There are approximately 27 million potential adult learners in Canada. Huge gains might reasonably be anticipated by creating a supportive environment linking on-line learners, who then invent new methods they share with their communities.

The Canada Foundation for Innovation and 2,000 new twenty-first century chairs for research excellence are helping to boost this marriage of technology with human knowledge.

The Canadian way – an early adopter

Dr Mike Binder, Assistant Deputy Minister, Spectrum, Information Technologies and Telecommunications, at Industry Canada, talks about the early days of Canada's Information Highway, in 1989, when media often referred to it as 'the information Hypeway!'

As early as 1994, the Government of Canada made a commitment to develop a Canadian Information highway strategy. An advisory council, composed of thirty members, spent 15 months designing over 200 recommendations, guided by three compelling objectives:

- Creating jobs through related innovation and investment in Canada
- Reinforcing Canadian sovereignty and cultural identity
- Ensuring universal access for citizens at a reasonable cost.

Emerging from this agenda was a view that support for lifelong learning should be a key design element of Canada's information highway strategy.

In Canada, Dr Binder has created a SchoolNet advisory board with deputy ministers of Education from provincial governments. School boards and unions came to a '*Eureka!*' consensus very rapidly, seeing that Newfoundland physics programmes and British Columbia physics programs were fundamentally the same. They are now working together to create a market for Canadian textbooks on-line. In Canada, we spend some $55 billion a year on educating our students, so educators will have many other '*Eureka*' moments, as we strengthen a learning society approach in this country.

Today, there is wide recognition that the economic miracle we are witnessing is emerging from the connected economy (Roth and Pecaut 2000), with nearly 50 per cent of Canadians having home connection to the internet and a large majority of businesses also reporting access.

Excavating diamonds in the rough

Few organisations in the Canadian federal firmament understand better than Natural Resources Canada (NRCAN) that knowledge is created and applied in a community of learners (National Resources Canada 2000). A federal department populated by scientists and other talented professionals, the practitioners in NRCAN are honing the human skills, relationships, technologies and communities of practice required to capture emerging knowledge, rather than simply capturing existing knowledge.

Just as a person can be identified by their own unique DNA, federal departments can be differentiated and uniquely identified by their organisational culture and results. Within this context, NRCAN has taken an innovative approach to being a knowledge leader.

Dr Peter Harrison, the Deputy Minister of NRCAN, notes that his department is in a very real way a 'best-kept secret'. His department directs natural resource policy decisions, delivers programmes for Canadians, operating with a health, safety and well-being mission that encompasses economic, social and environmental interests. Unless there is a serious earthquake or landslide, the 'no news is good news' message applies for a number of his knowledge-based programmes. However, without the scientific knowledge and industrial research generated by NRCAN in areas of sustainable development, ocean mapping, climate change, mining, forestry and nuclear power, for example, the private sector in Canada would be significantly less informed and focused in its business development.

Unlike the private sector, the geophysics knowledge that NRCAN possesses from exploring Canada's western basin, for example, is publicly available via its CANMET programs and websites. The challenge, Dr Harrison notes, is meeting the demands of a domestic and global clientele whose appetite for resource-based scientific advice, information and products is insatiable. This demand has grown with the development of Canada's North, in particular, with the creation of the new territory of Nunavut. It took 5 years alone to survey Canada's Far North.

Over hundreds of years, surveying land had changed little. Until recently, surveyors would be sent out with traverses to cover 15 to 20 km per day. Now surveyors enter information in digital form into a hand-held computer, load it up into a DGPS (digital global positioning satellite system), then this is descrambled and downloaded into a laptop computer and stored digitally, harmonising findings on the ground with satellite and aerial survey data.

What would normally have taken a decade to map can be done in months or a year at most. Now a claim for mining can be staked in very short order, on-line. This technology and the resulting knowledge have also been made available by NRCAN to the surrounding community members and aboriginal leaders.

NRCAN's scientists and explorers were in the Klondike before the Klondike was formed and in the Northwest Territories, identifying diamond formations before mines were established. Dr Harrison, Patricia McDowell, and their colleagues, are some of Canada's nation-builders.

Canada's Policy Research Initiative

The Government of Canada established the Policy Research Initiative (Government of Canada 2000) just over 4 years ago. The Initiative is strengthening the federal policy research capacity, with emphasis on medium to long-term policy issues facing the country. Laura Chapman, who heads the PRI, speaks passionately of the partnerships they have created with leading academics in Canada, with individual researchers in the private sector and with policy research specialists federally. They have created communities of knowledge and of interest around key public policy themes. Some of these thematic research projects appear on their website, where they receive over 2 million visits per year. This enthusiastic and clearly engaged research community rivals the kind of traffic that is seen on premium value commercial sites.

Chapman observes that federal research tends to be driven by short time lines and specific knowledge for a specific policy or program. Academic research timelines are much more discretionary and the research tends to be curiosity-driven. Marrying the two worlds has created some very interesting 'offspring' and has clearly generated an interest in wider communities.

However, the biggest challenge in achieving this marriage has been one of creating transdisciplinary understanding. Sociologists and economists, for example, have traditionally demonstrated little understanding of one another's language or world perspectives. At the heart of the work Laura Chapman and her team are undertaking is a desire to integrate disciplinary knowledge and to engage senior officials in a strategic harvesting of valuable knowledge.

Chapman emphasises that a major source of the PRI's success is due to the unique environment in which they work, the benefits accruing from being part of a knowledge-rich community of 7,000 people who have a relationship with the PRI, and who contribute to public policy formulation.

The Leadership Network

Mary Gusella, the Deputy Minister of Canada's Leadership Network (TLN), is leading another extraordinary experiment emanating from the Government of Canada. Her organisation is applying a new vision with regard to networks of leaders at all levels for Canada's public service. TLN is about investment by the corporate system in experimenting in new ways to deliver key services in the modern human resources management world. She notes that PS managers are not accustomed to declaring experimentation as an alternative vision to doing the old things in the old ways. She further rejects the traditional system that rewards technocrats and old-style crisis managers. Her definition of new-style crisis management means having leaders whose decisions deposit us gently ahead of issues.

Gusella and her team are developing a leadership laboratory that invites leaders to create conceptual frameworks to meet their business and leadership challenges. The Leadership Network represents a 'safe haven' where leaders can begin to see an ethic of care in action, where mentoring occurs and is prioritised as a developmental activity. Simply put, the philosophy is that if we care for a leader, then they will learn how to care for others. Gusella asserts that it makes no sense at all to say people have financial accountability but little or no accountability for developing other human beings. She begins with the premise that leaders not only want to do the best that they can do, but that they will raise the bar behaviourally and ethically, when given the right support and the opportunity to do so.

Often, private and public sector leaders betray an Industrial Age legacy base when they speak of employee retention. This has become something of a rallying cry for leaders competing for talented and scarce knowledge workers. Gusella, it can be argued, approaches the issue of leadership from the other end of the telescope – by creating a supportive work environment where employees and leaders know that their organisation cares about them. With the leadership incubator Gusella and her small band of revolutionaries are intent on constructing, the issue of retention becomes irrelevant. People stay because they choose to do so – an important lesson for any modern organisation.

A values transfusion

Bob Ward, also based within TLN, speaks of transfusing the whole PS with values and knowledge. He notes that any organisation seeking to adopt modern practices can not do so if its leaders are not what he calls 'a modern board of directors'. Citing as an example the Muskoka region of Ontario, where many of even the smallest and most humble dwellings may boast a satellite dish, miles away from the hue and cry of busy cities, Ward observes that our Canadian citizens are incredibly well-plugged into public policy issues. He suggests that governments are moving slowly away from 'power' relationships into relationships with citizenry focused on applied learning and a mutual value exchange.

We get, he emphasises, exactly what we deserve in the PS of Canada. 'Modern leaders, good people, will always find a new place to be modern', he argues, as he advocates a different way of measuring 'success' for leaders. Ward points out that many of the newcomers to the PS that he has working with his team in TLN understand that if you are not experimenting, then you are not learning or innovating.

A community of leaders as learners

Tom Stewart, a TLN leader, has been engaged in developing the collective management framework for the assistant deputy minister (ADM) community.

Prior to the collective management model being instituted, in 1996, Stewart observes that 82 per cent of ADMs had been promoted via their own department and did not always possess diverse experience. Now, 50 per cent of ADMs are appointed with transdisciplinary experience acquired in many settings. Currently, of the 250 ADMs in the PS in any 1 year, fully one-third are moving into or around the government, so there is an opportunity for leadership development and change. These new leaders, Tom Stewart suggests, are actively acquiring self-knowledge in a very different way from their predecessors as they partner with mentors, executive coaches and others who help them with their self-mastery and ability to work in teams and human networks.

Also within TLN, Mary Crescenzi is creating website-based communities of leaders who are learning about the art of living leadership at all levels of the PS. By connecting federal leaders, from Nunavut to Newfoundland, participating leaders are learning about the work of public servants via 'a day in the life of public servant' (Leadership Network 2000) business challenge features, chat forums and study groups. With 1.5 million hits per month, these websites have an active membership that represents an immense resource of knowledge and experience.

The next stage of this work sees Crescenzi and her team working with federal regional councils to develop a virtual network prototype which will provide a platform for leaders at all levels to gather electronically to meet and exchange information with members within their own community. The philosophy behind these sites and related webcasts has been to provide enabling tools to help knowledge-based communities nurture their own leadership and to access expert advice from their colleagues in real time. They have created a national advisory group to help design the site's content in each region of the country for a nationwide launch in the spring of 2001.

The Task Force on an Inclusive Public Service

Dr Janet Smith, the intrepid Deputy Minister head of the Task Force on an Inclusive Public Service, was given the daunting task, less than 2 years ago, of enrolling federal public servants in the creation of an inclusive PS and a very different future. She and her 3,000 activists decided to tackle some of the most basic assumptions underlying the public service culture.

Dr Smith started with the 'leadership efficiency' argument, an inherent part of the water we swim in, culturally speaking. This argument would have us believe that people at the top of organisations know more than those at the bottom. The Task Force decided at the outset that people all through the PS are capable of exercising leadership and undertook their work accordingly.

Many of the private sector leaders with whom the TF consulted applauded this approach to being inclusive but noted that there were some huge risks associated with empowering people fully. The Task Force rejected the established efficiency model as being inadequate for the challenges of a modern workplace where innovation and intelligent risk-taking at all levels go hand-in-hand. As Smith notes:

> If you think about where we've come from and the history of corporations, borrowing from military and church traditions, we've been captivated with a time and motion model. This means that routine tasks could be done in a specified time period and that we could calculate the related human labour required.

Managers in machine bureaucracies often regarded people as being interchangeable. Further, Smith believes that we are still in awe of this machine model, with too many of our measurement indicators predicated on input and output measures that do little to improve the quality of human life. She argues, 'Our work today is invariably about making choices minute by minute. Managers who are still trying to be efficiency leaders will undoubtedly have people throwing up their hands and saying "I can't do it!"'. It is from precisely these pressures that Smith concludes that we have been driven to a new model of knowledge creation and of leadership, because there is nowhere else to go.

As the head of the TF, Dr Smith helped design a world-class diversity instrument that measures how diverse a workplace is relative to where its employees say it needs to be. She also devised training programmes and live broadcasts with thousands of public servants that enabled us to commit to changes to create a more diverse and supportive workplace. Dr Smith paints a picture of what the PS will look like 3 years from now, if we've achieved the creation of an inclusive workplace. It will be, she argues, a place where people own the circumstances of their workplace. If they see something that is not working well, people will assume the responsibility for making this work well. There will be no more 'big mysteries', Smith says, when we all agree something is irretrievably broken and fail to act to remedy the situation. Power, we conclude, is derived from the human capacity for action, not from authority. She adds that we will no longer simply seek to recruit 'people like us', as part of a self-reinforcing system, but that we will hire people from all backgrounds. Unlike a closed system where we do not see new ideas because there is no one new to actively question our world view, we will live in a world where much more is being questioned, as a legitimate way of improving our workplace, 'we must come clean on this! We will never be a learning organisation until we embrace intelligent risks, diverse ideas and unconventional employees (shift disturbers), and see breakdowns as a way of achieving growth'.

A recipe for knowledge creation – The Association for Professional Executives of the Public Service of Canada (APEX)

APEX is the advocate of the interests of public service executives and a committed promoter of professionalism and management excellence. It is a network of more than 3,000 and executives and middle managers aspiring to create a more vibrant, challenging and responsible public service. Pierre DeBlois, the Executive Director of APEX, argues that their formula is simple: use the accumulated knowledge and experience, the collective wisdom and the vision of all executives to formulate policy and process within the PS.

> Many people used to think that the management team of the public service was just the DM community and the central agencies – we have always believed that the team is in fact all the 3,200 executives of the public service. Our role is to ensure they have a voice and that they have opportunities to participate in creating the vision and making it happen.

The secret to knowledge creation and to intellectual stimulation, DeBlois believes, is bringing people together in small, informal groups to discuss issues of common interest:

> Create the right environment for people to be creative! Get together after hours, out of the office, whatever it takes to provide a relaxed atmosphere. Our approach has worked. APEX's consultations with a multitude of interested parties have invariably resulted in a forward-looking agenda that creates action leadership.

DeBlois believes a key litmus test for success is whether Canadians recognise the contribution of their public services. Gaining this level of recognition means having a public service, he believes, whose leadership governs with its 'heart', not simply with systems, procedures and calculators in hand. He notes we are learning to reinvent ourselves to respond to the needs of Canadian society and that we must continue to do so if we are to remain relevant. He cautions against vesting too many of our intellectual 'eggs in the basket of huge policy shops'. This caution is offered because one dominant stream of thinking, referred to by DeBlois as 'inbred' thought, may prevail and challenges coming from operational players who live in reality and the effects of policy changes on citizens can be ignored. In fact, good policy and programmes are usually the product of 'cross-fertilisation'.

Pierre DeBlois concludes that in a time-poor society, we react too often and stop to think too rarely. For him, leadership is clearly a form of authentic self-expression that, when shared with others, creates value-added for the benefit of our citizens and employees.

A view from Canada's first Chief Information Officer

Linda Lizotte-MacPherson, the federal government's first Chief Information Officer (CIO), recently returned to the private sector from which she had been temporarily seconded. As a thought leader and co-creator, with the federal CIO community and deputy ministers, in designing federal IT/IM programs and infrastructure, Lizotte-MacPherson understood that this new role was inherently about business service transformation. As an enabler and a translator, frequently explaining technology, her primary focus was on creating the human capacity to accompany and support technological progress. For example, when learning upon her arrival that 50 per cent of federal executives could potentially retire by 2003, this became a compelling case for going beyond the status quo and creating new PS capabilities and capacities.

The 'e-experience', Lizotte-MacPherson emphasises, means placing more emphasis on human behaviours, not less. Many commercial sector corporations she cites are seeking to employ anthropologists and psychologists to help them design higher-value human interactions on-line. Technology is, in effect, enhancing the substance of people's jobs and creating stronger human networks. The federal government, she notes, can also be a model user of technology and can enter into strategic partnerships with other levels of government, other sectors, for example, by conducting government procurement on-line. Lizotte-MacPherson underlines improvements in productivity, the availability of multi-level government information, and the ease of doing business with the government as three major benefits that will accrue from the Government-On-Line (GOL) programme, when it is fully implemented, by 2004 (Treasury Board Secretariat of Canada 2000). Celebrating successes, she strongly believes, also helped to maintain the momentum for these important initiatives and helped create a commitment to reporting publicly on achievements.

Knowledge partners in Canada's health information highway

Bill Pascal, recently appointed as the head of Canada's health information highway in Health Canada, speaks in compelling terms of the different expectations of various demographic groups in our society with respect to the health knowledge Health Canada is dispensing federally, on-line.

The younger cohort, he says, are asking us to 'show us your value' and are challenging us 'to do it quickly' when they connect with the federal government electronically. Older and middle cohorts believe in the need for good governance and see the federal government as an honest broker.

Pascal notes that Canadians are wary of the American health care system that is perceived as one for elites. We agree that the 'radio station' many are listening to in this context appears to be WIIFM or 'What's In It For Me!'

He further opines that what's made Canada's health care system strong and unique is our ability to balance the individual's well-being with the collective good and well-being.

As an example, he mentions their 'Telehealth' initiative, which provides multi-media and telephone, computer health services linking health care professionals with patients in remote areas of Canada. The federal government got involved in the creation of a health system, in the early part of this century, due to real asymmetry in the health system and because of the catastrophic costs of dealing with treatments. Treatment was often beyond people's means and in the days before a national health care system was established, medical professionals possessed specialised knowledge and the patient was not well-equipped to manage their own health. Today, by comparison, the health system has rebalanced the equation.

Patients come into doctors' offices, bearing medical reports extracted from internet sites, wanting to engage doctors in a shared partnership around health-care decisions. This is, as Pascal says, an incredibly interesting case study in how citizens are using new knowledge to reinvent how we conduct business.

The Royal Canadian Mounted Police

Canada's Royal Canadian Mounted Police (usually referred to as the RCMP) are a venerable public institution of which Canadians are justifiably proud. Since the RCMP function as a national police force across Canada, RCMP members have deep roots in every part of our society. The ability to see emerging patterns, to digest new knowledge and to apply it rapidly is being aggressively developed by the RCMP. Deputy Commissioner Eva Kmiecic and the Commissioner of the RCMP, Giuliani Zaccardelli, are committed to having the RCMP recognised as the premier police and law enforcement agency in the world.

An example of innovation within this venerable institution is that of the award-winning CAPRA operational policing model, developed by Dr Frum Himelfarb and her team, as one of the key intellectual assets of the RCMP. This learning and community policing model has provided a framework for improved client-centred policing that connects talented police officers with other knowledgeable officers and expert knowledge bases to better serve citizens.

Accessible to employees of the RCMP in 720 locations across Canada and internationally, the CAPRA model and the related on-line university programme have cut traditional training costs by, in some cases, approximately 50 per cent. CAPRA stands for clients, acquiring and analysing information, partnership, response and assessment. It is a unique operational model that allows RCMP employees to exercise any combination of service, protection, prevention, enforcement and alternative options, such as restorative justice, before or when a problem arises.

The RCMP's CAPRA model is accessible to any internet (http://www.rcmp-learning.org) user and guides RCMP employees through self-development with individualised instruction modules, suggested assignments and coaching opportunities, among other things. Core competencies are developed along with functional job requirements for new opportunities that people may aspire to perform.

The site has logged millions of visitors, with as many as 200,000 per month. Detectives from Scotland Yard, gendarmes from France, the FBI and members of social justice networks from around the globe have eagerly used this continuous learning treasure. Student-centred learning has replaced an instructor focus and there has been a shift from rules-based learning to applied values and judgement.

Dr. Himelfarb is most proud of the reorientation in thinking that this policing program represents. As a modern management and governance framework, enshrining principles of partnership, self-actualisation, continuous learning and social inclusion, it is an operational model that many organisations may aspire to. The feedback coming from officers in the field is its own best reward for Himelfarb and her dedicated team. Emergency response teams have avoided confrontations and RCMP officers have been able to employ restorative justice models because they have analysed situations within this new framework.

Values-based modern management

Frum Himelfarb shares a deeply moving story of a new constable working in the field who was able to deal sensitively with a suicide, as the result of what he had learned via the CAPRA model. The constable told Frum that he had learned to prevent problems from happening instead of waiting for a problem to unfold. Officers following these programs quickly learn that they should know their communities intimately and graduates of the CAPRA program have to complete a project in their community that corrects a problem or prevents one. They are then required to write a paper on it and to share the resulting knowledge gained. As Frum Himelfarb underlines, this is a very different way of applying public policy, where policies are informed by the community's experience, unique context and knowledge. However, Himelfarb is quick to acknowledge that the best RCMP officers had always done much of this intuitively so the model was a way of ordering this knowledge, making it readily available to all and embedding it.

More importantly, RCMP employees learn as almost second nature to ask 'what do I know, don't know, and where do I go for more information?' After each policing interaction they assess how their clients felt they did, identify any emerging patterns, learn how to prevent an incident from happening again and record this for their fellow learners.

Diversity and learning in teams is regarded as an intrinsic part of this model. Those interested in wire-tapping or evidentiary issues can link into a knowledgeable community of practice and find out what is relevant to their context. Himelfarb says her programmes are informed by and designed with her users' needs in mind. If officers spend 15 minutes on one part of the site at a time, then she designs that component for 15 minutes of targeted access. Some modules offer chat groups and opportunities for interaction and classroom time as a shared experience. In the hate crimes module, for example, instead of simple classroom instruction, with technical lectures, speakers from the Canadian Human Rights Commission, victims and others interact to discuss ethical issues in the context of the police profession, linking policy specialists with citizens and practitioners.

Traditional police forces have often been preoccupied with issues around the 'use of force' model and officer survival programs that, while necessary, were silent about citizens and managing incidents without force. CAPRA has changed the emphasis to de-escalating the use of force and using negotiation wherever possible. Experienced officers will tell you that their mouth is their best weapon in an incident. RCMP officers see their role as being one of ensuring public safety by using the least possible intervention for the least possible harm or damage. The Public Complaints Commission has applauded CAPRA's risk assessment model that teaches officers to assess the likelihood versus the extent of harm in the seven points of an investigation. The likelihood of officers responding calmly in an incident has meant the RCMP is succeeding more frequently in moving issues from high- to medium- to low-risk situations.

Dr Himelfarb modestly notes that this intervention model would never have worked without the active participation of field officers and even, initially, of some naysayers. 'Things that make sense' she says 'eventually sell themselves, as the members of the police community share their acquired knowledge.'

If imitation is the sincerest form of flattery, then the CAPRA model, which has already entered RCMP vocabulary, as in 'to CAPRICIZE' something, is world-class. The commission on policing in Northern Ireland, police forces throughout the USA and elsewhere are building elements of their supervisors' field officers' and detachment commanders' development around the RCMP CAPRA program.

Fairy godmother – Merlin for a day

In interviews undertaken in support of this chapter, each leader was asked to imagine they were fairy godmother or Merlin the wizard for a day and to discuss what they would do if they could change anything they wanted in the Government of Canada, the Public Service of Canada or our society more generally. What emerged was an extraordinary blueprint, I would argue, for government in the knowledge-based economy:

- Ensuring innovators are developed
- Looking at life sciences partnerships and organisations for new governance models
- Actively recruiting energetic, dynamic youth into the PS of Canada
- Connecting the world by computer to close the digital divide, thereby fostering world peace and prosperity
- teaching all nations how to benefit from technology, science and the internet
- Giving executives permission not to know everything and to feel comfortable admitting they are not omniscient
- Introducing the concept of coaching as a management style and way of being
- Changing our risk/accountability model to one for the twenty-first century
- Ensuring knowledge sharing
- Actively developing all knowledge workers, not just star performers
- Focusing on an agenda for social cohesion so that we can liberate human potential and realise the strength in diversity
- Building trust-based relationships with aboriginal communities
- Eliminating fear in the workplace
- Focusing on public service values and what we need to do to achieve the public good, to create a burning sense of purpose and clarity for public servants; learning becomes a by-product of an 'electric passion' to serve Canadians
- Making it illegal to buy/construct things that create a barrier for the disabled and impede their full participation in our society
- Leaders who are learners committing to creativity, innovation and service, from which everything else would flow
- Establishing the twenty-first century as the Golden Age of new knowledge leadership.

Clear vision

While no one has suggested that Canada is a perfect, 'enchanted kingdom', you will undoubtedly have sensed in this whirlwind journey, the 'magic' of human genius and spirit at work. In our harsh, northern climate, where life has often been about shared survival and growth, we are continuing a knowledge journey that represents improved human well-being, on our own terms.

Acknowledgements

The author wishes to thank all those who contributed to this chapter. In particular she would like to pay a very special tribute to Dr Alexander Himelfarb, The Honourable Jocelyne Bourgon, Frank Claydon, Carole Swan, Richard Neville and Shalini Anand for providing inspiration and support for this project. Warm thanks are owed to Greg O'Brien for his longer-term role in the author's life.

References

Association of Professional Executives of Canada. (2000) Ottawa. Online. Available HTTP: http://www.apex.gc.ca/

Bourgon, J., The Hon. (1999) 'Keynote address by Jocelyne Bourgon, President, Canadian Centre for Management Development at the Technology in Government Week'. 19 October 1999: Ottawa, Canada.

Bourgon, J., The Hon. (2000) 'A public service learning organization: from coast to coast to coast, a policy discussion paper', Ottawa: Government of Canada.

Canadian Heritage (2000) Ottawa. Online. Available HTTP: http://www.pch.gc.ca (26 October 2000).

Canadian Institutes of Health Research. (2000) Ottawa. Online. Available HTTP: http://www.cihr.ca/whats_new/latest_info/newsmenu_l.shtml (26 October 2000).

Cappe, M., The Hon. (2000a). 'Report to the Prime Minister on the Public Service of Canada, from the Clerk of the Privy Council of Canada and Head of the Public Service', Ottawa: Government of Canada, March 31, 2000.

Cappe, M., The Hon. (2000b) 'Opening address by the Clerk of the Privy Council – APEX Symposium, May 31, 2000, Ottawa: Government of Canada.

Chrétien, J. (2000) 'Prime Minister's Address to a Team Canada Atlantic Business luncheon, 8 May 2000', Boston, Massachusetts.

Conference Board of Canada (2000) 'Collaborating for Innovation – 2nd Annual Innovation Report', Ottawa: Conference Board of Canada.

Health Canada (2000) Ottawa: Canada. Online. Available HTTP: http://www.hc-sc.gc.ca http://www.hc-sc.gc.ca (10 January 2001).

House of Commons, Standing Committee on Industry (2000) Ottawa: Canada. Online. Available HTTP: http://www.parl.gc.ca (10 January 2001).

Industry Canada (1999a) 'Community Access Program – Proposal Guide', Ottawa: Industry Canada. Online. Available HTTP: http://cap.ic.gc.ca (10 January 2001).

Industry Canada (1999b) 'The SchoolNet Grassroots National Campaign – Building a Strong Future for Canada', Ottawa: Industry Canada. Online. Available HTTP: http://ic.gc.ca (10 January 2001).

Leadership Network (2000) 'A Day in the Life of the Public Service of Canada', Ottawa: Minister of Public Works and Government Services. Online. Available HTTP: http://leadership.gc.ca

Martin, P., The Hon. (2000a) 'Federal Budget Speech', 28 February 2000, Ottawa, Tabled in the House of Commons, Government of Canada.

Martin, P., The Hon. (2000b) 'Speech to the Toronto Board of Trade', 14 September 2000, Toronto. Online. Available HTTP: http://www.fin.gc.ca

Massé, M., The Hon. (2000) 'Canada in the World, Speech to the APEX Symposium', 31 May 2000. Ottawa.

National Resources Canada (2000) Ottawa: NRC. Online. Available HTTP: http://www.nrcan.gc.ca/

Government of Canada (2000) 'Policy Research Initiative', Ottawa: Government of Canada. Online. Available HTTP: http://policyresearch.gc.ca/

Roth, J. and Pecaut, D. (2000) 'Fast Forward: Accelerating Canada's Leadership in the Internet Economy – Report of the Canadian E-Business Opportunities Roundtable, January 2000', Ottawa: Canada: Canadian E-Business Opportunities Roundtable.

Royal Canadian Mounted Police (2000) 'CAPRA', Ottawa: Royal Canadian Mounted Police. Online. Available HTTP: http://www.rcmp-learning.org

Tait, J. C. (original 1996; reprint 2000) 'A Strong Foundation. Report of the Task Force on Public Service Values and Ethics', Ottawa: Canadian Centre for Management Development.

Tibbetts, J. (2000) 'High court sees need for high-tech judges', *The Ottawa Citizen*, 23 August 2000; www.ottawacitizen.com

Treasury Board Secretariat of Canada (2000) 'Government On-Line Initiative', Ottawa: Treasury Board Secretariat. Online. Available HTTP:http://www.gol-ged.gc.ca

Treasury Board Secretariat of Canada (2000) 'Results for Canadians – A Management Framework for the Government of Canada', Ottawa: Treasury Board Secretariat. Online. Available HTTP: http://www.tbs-sct.gc.ca

Treasury Board Secretariat (2000) 'Task Force on an Inclusive Public Service 2000 @ 2000', Ottawa: Treasury Board Secretariat. Online. Available HTTP: http://www.tbs-sct.gc.ca/inclusive

Chapter 6

Reasoned strategy or leap of faith?

Knowledge management-led cultural change in Canadian public services

Susan Pollonetsky

Introduction

The underpinning hypothesis of the research presented in this chapter is the view that making knowledge management (KM) work in the public sector requires a leap of faith for all those involved. It also requires some degree of shared conviction at all levels of the organisation, but most critically at senior levels, that knowledge, both tacit and explicit can be transferred and shared profitably through the generation of new knowledge. It is through this process that real value may accrue in terms of leveraging the capacity of an organisation to be both effective and innovative in their area of operation.

The findings and discussion in this chapter are based on a small key informant survey of leading public and private sector executives and social scientists. Key research questions emerged from the desire to establish from the perspective of a range of contributors, their views on the author's assertion that knowledge management is generally perceived as representing an uphill climb in most complex organisations. However, it is rendered even more difficult in the public sector, because traditionally public services are geared more towards the generation and preservation of information silos, rather than knowledge sharing and dissemination.

The sense of urgency or burning platform that is present in private enterprise to demonstrate profitability has been notably absent from the Canadian public sector. On the other hand, the increasing use of the terminology of efficiency, effectiveness and fiscal prudence, as well as emphasis on the bottom line, provides evidence that there are clearly drivers to introduce and embed KM practices across government services.

Methodology

Interviews were conducted with both public and private sector executives and leaders via a key informant survey carried out in the summer and early fall of 2000. With two exceptions dictated by distance and inclement weather, all interviews were conducted in person.

While each interview was by design open-ended, the basic premise that guided my enquiries is that organisational culture matters to knowledge management; that the cultural context is the key determinant for its successful adoption and implementation.

Key questions posed to each person interviewed attempted to elicit ways and means to promote collaboration, open knowledge sharing environments, eliminate information silos and leverage knowledge assets in the public service. Each interviewee was asked to provide views on the following areas:

- Is culture amenable to change?
- How do you set about changing culture?
- Can you train or influence people to become collaborative knowledge sharers?
- Is there an optimal culture for introducing knowledge management (KM) into an organisation?
- What are some of the key determinants for promoting culture change?
- What sorts of levers/rewards and incentives are needed and finally, are there limitations on achieving change?

Developing a new understanding of the organisation

At the commencement of this research there was a desire to identify core components of organisational culture which could, if identified and understood, be managed in such a way as to facilitate the absorption of KM into the public service environment. At the end of the investigation it was far from proven that there was one clear answer to the question of how to create conditions or change corporate culture to support KM. However, a clear theme emerging through all of the investigations was perhaps best articulated by Dr Debra Wallace, Adjunct Faculty at the Faculty of Information Science, University of Toronto, 'culture trumps everything'. This is the clear focus of the work discussed in this chapter.

A rudimentary review of the study of organisational behaviour and theory reveals that it has emerged as something that is treated primarily as a scientific discipline – scientific in the sense that the term suggests an approach that is essentially mechanistic and focused upon ensuring replication of practice. Thus, classic organisational theory tended to be overtly mechanistic in approach and appeared to ignore or minimise the importance of human factors in the functioning of the organisation. A well-run organisation was compared to a well-oiled machine or in the words of organisational theorists such as William Bergquist, 'functioned like a carefully crafted Swiss watch' (Robinson Hickman 1998: 37). If things did not run smoothly there was no need to look much further than problems with the algorithm. There was much discussion of the ideal span of control for managers and the theory of the firm and much less concern with values and beliefs embedded in the firm.

Today however, there is a clear re-awakening that the most important determinant of an organisation's wealth is its people and their most significant contribution to the firm is the application of their knowledge to the firm. This renaissance of the value of the individual in the context of the organisation is one of the key drivers in knowledge management and it explains, in part, a heightened interest in studying organisational or corporate culture. After all, it is important to ask, once the lights are turned off and everyone has gone home, do you have an organisation or do you simply have real estate?

In key knowledge management literature, this emphasis on the valuation of the human element in knowledge transfer is dealt with in a variety of ways, directly and indirectly. There is evidence that it is the momentum behind the effort to measure intangible assets, such as intellectual capital and even relationship capital, that is leading to the emergence of a consensus that regards the prioritisation of knowledge transfer within organisations and the emergence of a new type of corporate culture, as being inextricably linked.

In response to the often-posed question, 'where are we heading?', the short answer is that to understand and influence culture change to support knowledge management whether it is in the private sector or the public sector, there is a need to look at views of corporate culture, necessary conditions for culture to change as well as barriers to culture change. This knowledge will then allow us to influence or direct such change through the use of various instruments and levers, and policies and incentives. Meaningful culture change, this research suggests, does not require possession of limitless resources. In the words of an interviewee, Jocelyne Bourgon, president of the Canadian Centre for Management Development who served as Canada's first female clerk of the Privy Council, 'Scarcity is the basis from which you manage great change'.

Views of corporate culture: part one

Divergent opinions exist about corporate culture. To some, it is somewhat of an oxymoron like the term 'jumbo shrimp'. Yet, all organisations do have a unique culture. Indeed if one were to ask six different organisational effectiveness consultants what constitutes corporate culture, it is likely that at least twelve different definitions would be proffered. As Marvin Bower a former McKinsey consulting firm executive stated, in reference to corporate culture, 'it's the way we do things around here . . .' (Robinson Hickman 1998: 26).

Thus it seems certain that corporate culture reflects the values and behaviours of people within the organisation. In Pottruck and Pearce's work, *Clicks and Mortar and Passion Driven Growth in an internet-Driven World*, the authors regard corporate culture as the unwritten rules and norms that are adhered to, as well as the informal and formal networks of decision making. Although these norms are founded on a set of shared values and can be formalised, they are rarely part of the regulations. Corporate culture in their analysis is defined as:

> ... a set of values, a common language and all the action that makes the values real. Values are the non-negotiable tenets against which we measure the worthiness of our choices. ... Accordingly, the values inherent in a culture are the basis for creating meaning for those who live and work in it. Values do not always dictate our behaviour but they do form the basis for our judgement of the worthiness of that behaviour.
>
> (Pottruck and Pearce 2000: 135)

Corporate culture in their view is purposive, rather than accidental, 'building culture is deliberate and difficult. ... It is at is heart, a thoughtful and lasting endeavour that starts with defining what is most important to us at the core.' (Pottruck and Pearce 2000: 45).

In *The New Work Culture*, Phillip Harris argues that 'an organisation's culture can help to turn its people on or off. That is, it can energise personnel, so that they accomplish, achieve and produce, or it can undermine employee morale, so that they are apathetic, uninvolved and unproductive' (Harris 1998: 32).

Ultimately, corporate culture can be elusive in its definition, but to overlook its significance can be a painful and expensive mistake for a public or private sector enterprise, large or small. In the context of introducing or embedding KM practices in the organisation, to misunderstand its importance is usually a recipe for failure.

How important is corporate culture to knowledge management?

Leading KM theorists and practitioners such as Thomas Davenport and Lawrence Prusak see corporate culture as being *the* determining factor in enabling KM to take root within the organisation, regardless of its sector of operation. In their recent book *Working Knowledge* (1998), they cite a number of key factors that inhibit the creation of a climate favourable to knowledge transfer within organisations. They considered a number of different case studies as they investigated the culture of knowledge transfer and what impeded knowledge transfer and found several key variables or inhibitors. In their analysis, what seemed to undermine the creation of more favourable conditions for transferring knowledge were:

- A lack of trust
- Different cultures
- Different vocabularies

- Conflicting frames of reference
- Lack of time and venues to hold meetings
- Narrow or restrictive ideas of productive work, disincentives built into rewards and recognition structures
- Rewards going to knowledge or topic owners
- intolerance within the organisation for mistakes or a need for help.

Among the experts and other knowledge management practitioners consulted for this research, there was a consensus that this cluster of 'KM inhibiting variables' comprised primary obstacles that would need to be surmounted in order to change the corporate culture.

If it is true that knowledge management presupposes new ways of working, sharing knowledge and collaborating across organisations, then we must understand the current complexities of public service environment as a first step in developing new, more coherent ways of working together. The choice of levers or instruments to support collaborative knowledge sharing, in this context, will also depend to a large extent on successfully identifying inherent views of organisational culture within the public service domain. As an interviewee for this research, David Zussman, President of the Public Policy Forum argues 'knowledge sharing is a strategic action, technology is an enabler for knowledge management, but cultural influences are strong and ultimately, KM needs people to act differently'.

Views of culture change: part two

In order to better understand the dynamics of culture change, a crucial first question posed to everyone interviewed was, did they see culture as being amenable to change or influence, or was it something that could in fact be managed, directed or shaped? Responses tended to fall into two categories: category 1: culture is ultimately changeable using active measures or category 2: culture cannot really be controlled but can be influenced indirectly. Nearly all agreed that organisational or corporate culture is amenable to change with appropriate rewards and incentives, modelling behaviours and visible buy-in or support from senior management, although there were significantly different opinions as to the rate and extent of changes that could be expected.

Category one: culture is ultimately changeable

Those who stated that they believed that culture is ultimately malleable or changeable tended to be very positive in their world view, technological determinists or both. According to Carole Swan, Associate Secretary, Treasury Board of Canada Secretariat, corporate culture is definitely changeable, through the use of different levers. A key question for her was do you change behaviour or ideas? Pragmatically, she also pointed to the fact that sometimes we do not have the luxury of time to wait for directional changes.

In many respects, the Treasury Board of Canada Secretariat can be seen as a microcosm of the wider public service arena. In the early 1990s, people were very much inward looking, focusing on their business alone in a way that was not ultimately beneficial to promoting knowledge sharing. Even if people were motivated to work in a more collaborative fashion, there were fewer cultural supports/rewards or any obvious recognition to promote more horizontal work styles.

Ms. Swan observed that the organisation is beginning to recognise the huge advantage of collaboration and co-operation but that there remains a need to have systems and approaches to re-invigorate such things as ensuring that the emphasis upon working in teams retains energy and focus. Changing the way in which the Secretariat works clearly demands time and requires appropriate incentives and rewards. As a large complex organisation, in common with many others in the public service domain, it is not known for its nimbleness. The very nature of the work, an imperative to be seen to be serving the public interest and the general variability of other political factors does preclude an organisation of this complexity from being naturally agile in approach.

As the administrative arm of the Treasury Board, the Secretariat has a dual mandate: to support the Treasury Board as a committee of ministers, and to fulfil the statutory responsibilities of a central government agency. It is headed by a secretary-comptroller general, Frank Claydon, who reports to the President of the Treasury Board, an elected Member of Parliament and cabinet minister, Lucienne Robillard. The Secretariat recommends and provides advice to the Treasury Board on policies, directives, regulations and programme expenditure proposals with respect to the management of the government's financial, human and material resources. Its responsibilities for the general management of the government affect initiatives, issues and activities that cut across all policy sectors managed by twenty-two operating departments and some 100 other organisational entities.

The Secretariat also supports the Treasury Board in its role as the general manager and employer of the public service. The main areas of activity in the central administration of the public service cover expenditure management, personnel management, financial and information management, as well as internal administration of the Treasury Board of Canada Secretariat including internal executive direction provided to the Secretariat, including information, financial, personnel and administrative services. The complexity of the Secretariat's role and responsibilities and the concomitant machinery that is necessary to support its work can easily be seen as a mitigating force affecting an organisation's ability to become more agile and nimble.

Swan also observes that by changing rewards and incentives, including developing some non-remunerative, yet valued incentives such as recognition, as well as developing some incentives to salary structure, will serve to reinforce more of the behaviours that are desired become embedded in the work place.

Richard Neville, Deputy Comptroller General, comptrollership branch, Treasury Board Secretariat also acknowledges that although the perfect culture is not evident in government nor are necessarily all of the elements in place in order change the (corporate) culture, he believes that this can in fact be done. Like Swan, he says it is possible to put levers into place, including recruiting the right people, and having the equipment and technology in place. Even such things as having personal computers at home, will help shift attitudes and approaches to work. Essentially, in his view, it is possible to move culture, by changing management practices and the organisational environment.

When asked about the impact of technology on organisations, Neville felt that on balance it does exert a significant influence. But in and of itself, it does not change everything. From his vantage point, by far the fastest route to influence culture is to bring people into one's organisation that possess 'broader horizons'.

For Lynn MacFarlane, the Associate Chief Human Resources Officer at the Treasury Board of Canada Secretariat, technology continues to play a huge role in ushering in profound culture change in the work place and in broader society. In her analysis, any discussion of cultural change must first recognise that our world is very different today and at the risk of over-stressing the impact of technology, she noted that several things hold true today which could not have been said even a few years ago:

- Nothing is secret
- Information cannot be managed nor contained
- Transparency is not only desirable, it is essential.

Creating a climate or the conditions conducive to knowledge sharing is not simply a 'nice to have', according to MacFarlane, it is a necessity and, further, it is in the greater public interest. The public interest is a powerful political force that is stronger than the individual or private interests leading her to conclude that, in this public service context, knowledge sharing is not a discretionary activity.

In MacFarlane's assessment, in the age of instantaneous communication, electronic eavesdropping, satellite imaging and night vision, nothing can be hidden and the more that institutions attempt to control and script events and manage issues, the more likely it is to unravel. The only option is transparency.

Conceding that technology changes preclude efforts to wield absolute control over our environment or culture and that human interventions have the capacity to affect culture change directly, suggests that in McFarlane's view, relatively profound cultural change can occur surprisingly quickly.

Another proponent of using active measures or interventions to direct cultural change is Dr Aidah Warah, a clinical psychologist and an organisational development specialist, with the National Research Council. She accepts that human cultures can be shaped, as human beings are capable of evolving and growing. By way of example she cites the use of less coercive powers in our human interactions on the whole, within society, we have developed legislative instruments to replace sticks. She also notes that culture tends to be self-reinforcing. People tend to hire and promote people who are like them. She believes that it is possible to move culture forward but this entails active leadership and even symbolic leadership, people who are willing to be 'spear carriers' or 'vanguards with stentorian voices'.

Michelle d'Auray, Chief Information Officer for the Government of Canada situates herself somewhere in the middle of the scale between those who believe that culture is not amenable to change and those who believe that it is, and that it can be directed and influenced. In terms of promoting knowledge sharing, d'Auray is more inclined to share everything within limited restrictions. She has been able to witness a good deal of cross-fertilisation of ideas through supported and constructive knowledge sharing between individuals. In her view, there will always be trade-offs between consultation and drawing out employee knowledge and the actual process of decision-making. Time or scarcity of valuable input can become the arbiter of how much effort should be made to achieve inclusive levels of input, prior to making a decision.

Denise Amyot, the Director General of Recruitment for the Public Service Commission of Canada also believes that cultural change is possible especially when you align the right things together: people, departments and the public: 'culture is a way of being, anyone can contribute to culture change if they are committed. How do you become committed? You need something that calls you.'

Amyot perceives a culture that has already changed at the Public Service Commission. People are talking more and more about values, as it seeks to transform itself from an organisation that has been primarily rules-based, to one that is values-based.

Culture is also a factor emanating from the people who make up the workplace. Amyot envisages enormous shifts in culture simply as a result of the impact of demographic changes. For example, 50 per cent of all executives currently employed will be eligible to retire by 2004. As many as 70 per cent of the current cohort could be gone by 2008. As younger people enter the public service with different values, attitudes to ownership of knowledge and working styles, culture shifts are likely to be even more pronounced.

Category two: culture cannot be controlled but it can be influenced indirectly

As was stated at the outset, for Deborah Wallace at the Faculty of Information Science, University of Toronto, 'culture trumps everything', including policy and vision within organisations, but it moves at a measured pace. 'A lot and at the same time, little has changed since Sir Francis Bacon stated that knowledge is power. Paradigms are shifting, but they are not moving overnight.'

Shaping culture is obviously a factor of endogenous and exogenous variables. Wallace notes that some private sector firms such as Hewlett Packard (HP) recognised that workplace culture has enormous impacts on how work is conducted, employee satisfaction and productivity. She reflects that for many years in the atrium at HP, during the mid-morning period between 10 a.m. and 10:30 a.m., free coffee and doughnuts have been served to all employees to promote informal conversations and knowledge exchange.

Wallace also notes that in new start-up companies, culture fit is very important; executives responsible for hiring are more worried about hiring for compatible attitudes rather than cognitive abilities. However, the essential nimbleness of the new start-up organisation is something that is largely alien to the public service environment, where, even when new agencies or organisations are created, they usually emerge from the amalgamation of legacy-based structures.

A number of interviewees expressed the view that culture is almost immune to persuasion or active manipulation and that human nature is by nature governed by self-interest. In the context of promoting a knowledge sharing culture, everything would depend on inducements to share and the opportunity costs of not sharing. Indeed, in some circles, the rallying cry about the need to examine cultural barriers or change culture was viewed with some suspicion, that it was more often a code for a lack of leadership.

What lends credence to this line of reasoning is the fact that open criticism of leadership or a lack thereof is rarely sanctioned in the private sector or in the public sector, except in specific circumstances such as visioning exercises, executive retreats and other exercises that are more or less contained or circumscribed. Otherwise, to criticise direction and leadership within one's own organisation can be seen as career limiting. On the other hand, by using culture change as the proxy for leadership, it can easily become the cloak for suggesting changes that involve culture, but begin and end with leadership.

Common wisdom would suggest that cultural change driven by visible leadership, will occur faster. That is not to say that it cannot evolve in the absence of strong direction, only that if the direction, depth and breadth of change is significant, then timeliness is also a key factor. That points to a need for leadership.

Others viewed culture as akin to happiness, that it is not an end in itself, only a by-product of doing the right thing. If people at all levels of the organisation and not just the leaders do the right thing, a changed and more flexible culture should inevitably follow. This would suggest that at most we can influence culture change indirectly, through action and deeds such as rewarding desired behaviours.

Evelyn Levine, Director General of Corporate Services for the National Library and Archives of Canada agreed that sharing of information and knowledge is critical, although in her experience sharing is not always a behaviour that has been valued or reinforced. Often knowledge is traded or bartered as a commodity, by people who act as 'information pimps'. For some people, information or knowledge is not to be exchanged freely. As a consequence, a type of corporate Social Darwinism takes root, survival of those most adept at leveraging their knowledge.

In other work environments where sharing is driven by a keen sense of and respect for interdependence and the necessity to not only survive, but thrive, there is a move toward 'co-opertition', that is co-operative competition. Not quite a utopian or broadly socialist vision of the sharing of knowledge but less than the capitalist or scarcity model of knowledge acquisition.

Creating a knowledge sharing culture is usually successful if the risk of sharing is encouraged within the organisation and the behaviour achieves beneficial results. Promoting knowledge sharing by edict as a way to force cultural change, has not been proven to be either effective or desirable.

Levine notes that although there is a lack of a sense of urgency for making sweeping changes to organisations to promote knowledge sharing, there are some important pressures within organisations that are driving cultural change, notably technology and interdependency. She further argues that:

> We are in the Juraassic Era and the great Ice Age (new technology) is here to stay. Technology will be the driver that ultimately moves us out of the Jurassic Era and will propel us forward. Technology will be the great glacier that separates the adaptable organisations that will prevail. New organisations that survive this age will be able to mutate quickly and adapt. People in these organisations (public and private) will either learn how to co-operate or stay on the sidelines . . .

Do the public services behave differently from the commercial sector with respect to cultural change?

With a career spanning both the public and the private sector, Gini Bethell believes that organisations, and the people within them, are amenable to change, with the appropriate incentives and models to follow. At the same time, she notes that private sector organisations are not as advanced as they are commonly perceived to be. They may have achieved some 'stepping stones', but not historic milestones en route to becoming transparent, agile, sharing, knowledge-management exemplars.

Dr Richard Van Loon, President of Carleton University with extensive experience in the public sector and academia also believes that there are fewer substantive differences in the way that public and private sector organisations use knowledge. He rejects any grand dichotomies between organisations in the public and private sector and notes that all senior managers regardless of their public or private provenance give just what they need in order to get what they need. Paraphrasing a veteran senior manager, Van Loon described 'potlach' behaviour, where people barter or trade information to maximise their competitive advantage. Seasoned managers, he argued, use a mental calculus when exchanging information:

- How much do I need to give away to get what I need?
- How much do I have to co-operate with others to get the most for my organisation?

This calculation, he feels, is not a prolonged action, it happens fast, and is based on intuitive knowledge.

In his assessment, perhaps the key difference between the public sector's adaptation to shifts in technology and the private sector's response can be seen in the pace of change. Unlike the corporate world, there is almost always a significant time lag in the public sector.

Arthur Kroeger, Chancellor of Carleton University and a former Deputy Minister of Employment and Immigration (a precursor of Human Resources Development Canada) agrees that technology diffusion may be slower in the public sector than in the private sector, although its impacts are likely to be more acute in public sector organisations. Members of Parliament in his estimation are most at risk simply because they are locked into established ways of doing things. The larger question becomes how to change the function of government machinery. In his estimation, there is currently evidence of a more connected pubic service environment, relatively engaged with the public/taxpayers. Members of Parliament and politicians across all strata of Canadian democracy, on the other hand, have to contend with the possibility of being by-passed in the emerging modes of operation. He argues 'there are risks inherent in change and changes in government (and governance) are political risks. Change agents within organisations are causing hierarchies to change. The challenge today is to be in a position to assess the full extent of these shifts and cultural changes.'

The downside of e-citizenry or direct democracy via instant polling and/ or on-line referendums could be the disintermediation of Members of Parliament from the machinery of government. This is a question yet to be answered by political scientists, but technically, one can envisage a society where the need for politicians could be obviated by fully implementing some of the knowledge gathering and knowledge dissemination technologies available today. In many respects this explains why knowledge management has come to be so feared or revered. For many it is regarded as the new watershed, perhaps the third industrial revolution because the very fact that how knowledge is shared and transferred ultimately has the potential to wrest the balance of power from the state and return it to the individual.

The importance of balancing asymmetries in knowledge was repeated in several discussions and as Michelle d'Auray, Chief Information Officer, Government of Canada notes, particularly in the age of information, it has become a key role for government, whether it is from the perspective of Environment Canada and its weather reports or sharing health and safety information to promote and protect the health and well-being of citizens.

In the opinion of Alan Nymark, Deputy Minister, Environment Canada, our interest in managing knowledge is not necessarily greater than it is in other sectors, especially private industry. On the other hand, because of asymmetries in knowledge, governments need to have collective ways of dealing with, transferring/sharing/communicating knowledge. To do this, we need to get smarter in managing knowledge internally as part of a global knowledge market. While certainly governments can take lessons in stream-lining, in becoming more open, transparent and coherent, the bottom line for government is different, it is always the public interest; balancing compet-ing interests to support the greatest number or those most in need in the most efficient and cost-effective way.

According to Nymark, currently much of the discussion in government is about absorbing the implications of the technology revolution and we are only really beginning to deal with more fundamental knowledge manage-ment issues. As recently as the 1980s, virtually no economists were looking at knowledge as capital. By the 1990s, knowledge began to be looked at as an endogenous rather than simply an exogenous variable. Government then started to look at the context of knowledge generation as influencing productivity growth and what instruments could influence this relationship. Whilst at policy level there is evidence that we are making strides in seeing knowledge as working capital in organisations, few would disagree that the momentum for valuing knowledge and measuring knowledge capital still rests largely with the private sector.

Views of technology

A dominant view in the evolution of culture is that technology will, and indeed already has, changed everything. In Van Loon's assessment, its impacts are far-reaching in organisations:

> What we tend to overlook is what do we do with this technology. The dilemma is that managers do not know what to do. Technology and

information technology in particular will support whatever managers define as important to do, including promoting a more open, knowledge-sharing culture, working more collaboratively, etc. To accomplish this we need to grapple with goals that managers have and those of the wider organisational context, which are often ill defined.

Although Van Loon agrees that the pace of change has been accelerating in the last 100 years, he refutes the notion that this is greater than any other period in history.

He also observes that technological change has had profound impacts not just on complex organisations, but on the very essence of statecraft. Looking at the more significant technologies developed and perfected in the century (the telephone, electricity, cars and telecommunications), regimes such as twentieth century totalitarianism could only have been supported by the evolution in communications networks.

Van Loon explained that without telephones and wiretapping devices omnipresent in 'Orwellian big brother is watching' states, they would not have been able to exert such strict controls over their citizenry during the cold war and afterwards. Further evolutions in the telecommunications industry meant that in an age of instant communications through television, and the advent of the internet, instead of big brother, the whole world was now watching and insular, oppressive, anti-democratic regimes would be placed at risk.

When we consider drivers of cultural change in organisations there are additional contextual factors to bear in mind that differentiate the public sector from the private sector. Knowledge is portable and people are also mobile. Companies may also come and go, but the public interest and safeguarding the public interest, is a constant. If we use uptake of technology as a proxy for how these respective organisations embrace cultural change, then it appears that change occurs more slowly in government.

Technology may determine the way we will interact, whether by email, in person, by fax, via a call centre for example, but it does not, of itself, determine the substance of our interactions and what we exchange by way of information. This is far more likely to vary with the underpinning philosophy of the organisation or service itself and the external factors of the environment in which it operates.

For Zussman, President of the Public Policy Forum, technology symbolises the ultimate twenty-first century paradox: technology has the potential to change everything or it can mean that you do everything the same way:

> The reality is that technology allows you to do things differently, if you choose to. Much will depend on characteristics of the organisations and of the people themselves. If you take a rigid structure and superimpose technology that enables sharing and collaboration it may not make that big a difference about how things get done. If you are not predisposed to

change, then technology is not a panacea that will make you think differently and act differently . . . much depends on attitudinal predisposition.

Similarly, Wallace does not see technology as the solution or the new standard, it is an enabler at best, or marginally an add-on. An example of technology at its very best is the way it has allowed scientists to create new pathways for collaboration and she cites such monumental endeavours as the mapping of the human gene or the human genome project. She also notes that the internet has raised some interesting issues around access and evaluation of content, 'we need to teach critical analysis but this could be one of the transitional things around the internet that may take at least a generation to absorb'.

However, not all the technology-driven changes can be presumed to be in the public interest. In the realm of governance, technology has already presented some serious challenges. Certain aspects of regulation will be or are already nearly impossible to enforce according to Dr Van Loon. He cites censorship of pornography as an example of an area of regulation that has been less available to governments within the last 30 years and probably will continue to be for some time to come.

No one can predict how far culture will evolve as a result of activities entirely attributable to technology although Kroeger, like many of his peers believes that the internet is beginning to change everything including not just how people retrieve information but how they assess information and knowledge. This in turn, he argues, will inevitably change behaviour within organisations. He cautions that much of the discourse around knowledge management in the context of creating and sharing knowledge is not really new. In his words, the evidence points to the contrary:

> In fact governments have been managing knowledge for years through horizontal management. At the same time, horizontality has boundaries. It can be in an agency's best interest not to provide a lot of information in order to reduce the risk of outside interference as well as to protect competitive advantage.

He further argues that, introducing new blood into public service organisations does not automatically presage major shifts in culture:

> In some ways hope about young people and different work styles can be somewhat misplaced. They can begin with fresh ideas, but their perspectives can age as they become entrenched within an organisation that is more traditional in its approach to sharing information and knowledge.

Within this context, technology can obviously be seen as an enabler for sharing knowledge and working collaboratively, but it is not a panacea. It is a tool and its utility ultimately rests with those who use it.

Critical success factors in achieving cultural change

If the challenge to introduce KM into public service organisations pivots on getting people to behave differently, there are some steps that can be taken to make this happen. The basic foundation, as the interview data collected for this chapter suggests, appears to be the existence of a healthy work environment. There are many recipes for success, but successful change initiatives must have most, if not all of the following elements in place.

Building trust

There are several must-haves or ingredients for effecting culture change, but the key ingredient for promoting a knowledge-sharing culture appears to be trust. Unless there is a high level of trust within an organisation, new initiatives and ways of working such as KM will only be grafted on and to borrow a medical metaphor, it will susceptible to graft-versus-host disease and the new initiative will not become successfully embedded.

Van Loon believes that levels of trust do not have to be at 100 per cent in the organisation, but there needs to be sufficient agreement about underpinning organisational goals. In order to have an impact on organisational culture or to change culture, typically managers will make a number of assessments.

Achievement of necessary levels of co-operation is generally possible with a top-down approach to change management. However, leadership at the top, from both executive post holders and from politicians, needs to demonstrate credible levels of buy in to this change in strategy or behaviour. They in turn will influence their own directors and other middle managers to adapt and adopt different practices. This may lead to the status of fixed organisational hierarchies being challenged, with more equitable and creatively capable public services emerging.

In Warah's assessment, seen from the vantage point of an organisational development specialist and a practising clinical psychologist, an important way to measure trust is to look at the overall resilience of the organisation. In order to do this, there is a need to explore how people deal with differences, how accepting they are of the diversity of ideas and how willing they are to deal with and learn from the unexpected. Other metrics include how much indirect communication there is and an assessment of core human interactions, so for example it is important to ask, do key individuals avoid direct communication and prefer to hide beyond the process orientation of traditional paper-based and meeting structures?

Building trust takes time. However as Dr Warah observes, once trust is broken, it is very difficult to rebuild. Use and abuse of trust within organisations is closely related to how people use power. You trust people who have shown benevolence, this shows that they do not intend to harm you.

She also notes that if we look at the nature of most relationships, that most are transactional or based on bartering. To build communities of interest people must generally be willing to contribute more than they can anticipate being able to take. However, too often people are conditioned to adopt a 'what's in it for me' stance:

> Our sense of self can either be narrowly or broadly defined. That in turn will make us interested in giving more or receiving more. Within organisations, benevolent caring people tend to be trusted more. In most organisations we will continue to have control mechanisms, but we must also maintain trust mechanisms.

Yet, how do we know when we are organisationally healthy? According to Dr Warah there is resilience and flexibility within the organisation and people feel fulfilled.

Part of learning how to co-operate and collaborate means building trust within organisations in Levine's assessment, 'if we consider another cultural norm in government, namely the culture of secrecy, there are obvious barriers to open sharing of information. We are working within a paradigm of operating strictly on a need to know basis.'

Thus, it seems clear that trust must be reciprocal and it must be built. It may take years to build up and an instant to erode. Open communication is a hedge against the corrosion of mistrust. As Amyot observes 'we need to cultivate ways to communicate better as individuals and within teams'.

Leadership

Executive buy-in and leadership are also at or near the top of the list of necessary conditions to promote a more open, knowledge-sharing culture within public service organisations according to data extracted from this key informant survey. For example, in Bourgon's analysis, leadership and management in any organisation are key influencers of cultural change capability. Strategic leadership, she argues, is about vision, commitment and enrolment. A task for management is to align people, power and purpose, in order to liberate ideas and promote knowledge transfer.

Further, Bourgon distinguishes between leaders and managers. The skills that they require are not always interchangeable. We need to ask who are the right leaders for the time? Managers in contrast tend to be the aligners, not necessarily the visionaries who she defines as those who are engaged in the process of creating a new public service reality.

Today we are faced with managing great change in an era of scarcity. Do we have enough leaders? Are they in the right place? In Bourgon's assessment, the simple answer is we do not need huge numbers, but we need the right people at the right moment in time, and at the right place, in order to manage breakthroughs.

Amyot agrees that buy-in and commitment is required of leaders at all levels but emphasises that it is most crucial, particularly at the assistant deputy minister and deputy minister level. To engage and motivate those around them, they need to demonstrate that they are living the culture change that they wish to see take root in their organisations. These leaders also need to understand from a behavioural standpoint, how to motivate those around them. As Warah observes:

> On one hand you want people who are not just populists, they must be empathetic enough to know what is needed. But you also need strong visionary leaders who can motivate others. Many people are ready and willing to follow new initiatives, but few are willing to assume risks . . .

Van Loon emphasises that leadership is also about building trust, 'leaders have to walk the talk, and consistency is important. As part of trust building, people have to be able to raise questions in an open environment without risk of repercussions.'

Wallace sums up the consensus view that merely saying the right things or paying lip service to people, values and culture is not sufficient. Diametrically opposed values and practices only lead to organisational dissonance. Within public service organisations, politicians and senior management clearly need to lead by example, setting an example from the top-down how to use knowledge and create new knowledge. In her experience, too often we see ineffective leaders; something of a cross between the classic management characterisation of the Peter Principle meets aspects of Social Darwinism discussed previously.

Behaviour changes

Zussman believes that knowledge management in the public sector depends on people acting differently. 'If you believe in it, if there is buy-in at levels of executive leadership, it can happen. Obviously, you need more of the key people doing this'. d'Auray agrees that a key driver for changing cultures is behavioural change. Technology has also had a real impact on how knowledge is transferred and shared. The internet, as an example has made knowledge hoarding that much more difficult, even in the face of natural proclivities.

From a psychological perspective, what lies at the heart of culture change is behavioural change, according to Warah:

> The challenge then becomes to look at what motivates behavioural change. Does it in fact make a difference if people make the right decision for the wrong reasons or for the right reasons? In many situations you need more than compliance.

In her assessment it is more likely that more profound shifts in culture will occur when people share knowledge because they want to rather than because they feel they have to.

Lasting (culture) change as Warah noted, 'can sometimes be reduced to the difference between compliance and commitment. Can you make believers out of non-believers? Fundamental, transformational change requires hard work, discipline and consistent effort. This is impossible if all you have is compliance.'

Amyot also notes that we often tend to recognise only the big things. Management's obligation is to recognise and reinforce other achievements and efforts. Culture will evolve as a result of efforts on several fronts including messages, leadership and the accountability regime. Individuals can be encouraged to share best practices and to do all of this, we need to nurture people in our organisations.

Restructure rewards/create incentives for culture change

Several different explanations were offered as to why rewards and incentives are so important in helping to shape culture, but everyone agreed to varying or lesser degrees, that they were needed. After a career in public service and now as Chancellor of Carleton University, Kroeger has seen and championed progressive changes in the public sector and the post-secondary education system, and is very familiar with culture change. His advice, drawn from many years of experience was simply stated as, 'you don't change culture by talking, you change culture by incentives'.

With this as a context, looking at the issues of culture change and KM, MacFarlane observes that traditionally, rewards and recognition do not go to the best managers of knowledge, they go to the best file managers. File management gets the kudos, not knowledge management. To change our approach to how we use knowledge within organisations we need to look at restructuring our rewards system and develop visible incentives that can serve to modify behaviours.

Reinforcing the behaviours you wish to see become entrenched requires a long term commitment and perseverance. Quoting a former head of the Canadian Broadcasting Corporation, Gerard Veilleux, Van Loon says, 'you only lose when you stop. Sooner or later the environment changes.'

Choosing the optimal incentives will vary according to the specific environment and the individuals concerned, but change agents and knowledge leaders in Van Loon's assessment need to show a type of opportunism in the most positive sense of that term, 'sometimes the worse things are, the better the likelihood of making positive changes'.

The consensus view emerging from this research suggests that given the appropriate rewards and incentives, and by rewarding desired behaviours rather than punishing or using sanctions to modify undesirable behaviours, eventually we will see organisational culture change.

Encourage collaboration

In Levine's experience, working in collaboration with partners outside government, necessitates sharing information, data and records, yet in her experience, sharing is not a value that is either valued or recognised. In Nymark's assessment, whilst it may seem desirable to work collaboratively, it is much easier at the initial ideas stage, and more difficult at the implementation stage. He cites the work of the Canadian government's Policy Research Initiative as a good example of nurturing collaboration. They have succeeded in getting people at the analytical level to work horizontally even before discussion of the in-depth policy issues take place. In addition, depending on the government department you happen to be in, the work across government for transition planning according to Nymark, serves as either an example of collaboration and knowledge sharing in some departments and agencies or working in secrecy. Ideas are more or less risky at different stages of the policy development process and our assessment of risk is uneven across organisations.

Nymark argues that it is important to self-evaluate from an organisational position the extent to which:

> . . . you encourage the flowers of innovation to grow when they are not immediately seen as crucial or important? Who is actually allowed to participate? When are ideas acceptable? Over time we need an agreement on what the scope is (within any organisation) for thinking outside the box. In other words, can we set out some guideposts for the learning process of an organisation.

Eva Kmeicic, Deputy Commissioner, Royal Canadian Mounted Police, agrees that to promote a more open, knowledge-sharing culture, there is a need to think differently and adjust machinery accordingly, in order to serve citizens and clients better. As part of ongoing efforts to behave as a knowledge-driven organisation, she believes it is critical that knowledge be visibly valued, invested in and subsequently marketed across the organisation. In practical terms this means recruit talent, train up, and improve the knowledge capital/stock of your organisation.

Kmeicic also advocates the building of communities of practice through support of special, visible projects. People will then take notice of different approaches to work styles and knowledge sharing. Through the act of combining best practices with globally focused leadership, you can then move organisational culture forward towards the ultimate goal of better knowledge sharing across the organisation.

Not surprisingly, in the private sector, the capacity to work collaboratively is regarded as a very desirable attribute. As the former Canadian CEO of EDS, now with the Australian EDS, Sheelagh Whittaker stated when questioned about the capacity for building networks, 'we don't hire for it, but we do promote for this as well as for curious minds. These are employees who are motivated to understand the environment in which they work.'

Different approaches to risk management/learning from mistakes

To enable new KM-focused organisations, management needs to accept that mistakes are a healthy part of risk management. As one seasoned senior mandarin recounted, 'as a government we are behind what we are telling others. We also tend to be risk averse, but our risk management approach is not an excuse for being dumb.'

Whittaker notes that there is a problem for governments in that they can become too mature in their outlook and too risk averse. There is a much smaller risk in closing things down that present risk or uncertainty, than to continue on an uncharted path.

How far then do organisations need to go in order to create fertile ground for better knowledge sharing and knowledge management? What steps need to be taken? Do we opt for risk taking versus risk management?

According to Whittaker, the key determinant for success and successful outcomes has more to do with commitment and risk profile than creativity or technological capability. Nymark agrees that governments can cultivate a capacity for being smart without being reckless:

> It is obvious that we cannot take the same risks as private industry, but we need to become more open to innovation. To do this means looking at how our institutions act, the skills inventory that they have and need to develop, their capacity to act horizontally, their ability to accept information and their willingness to share knowledge . . .

Conclusions

The opinions expressed in this chapter affirm that organisational culture is indeed amenable to change, with appropriate leadership, rewards and incentives, modelling behaviours and visible buy-in or support from senior management. To promote knowledge sharing, different levers can be used, but collaborative behaviours will not flourish on their own. To achieve this we will need to revisit how we recognise knowledge sharing within our organisations. This in turn needs to be incorporated into our assessments and remuneration packages for employees at all levels.

However, over and above a mechanistic approach to fixing rewards and incentives there is strong consensus that embedding knowledge sharing and harvesting of knowledge within the public sector represents a major values and paradigm shift, that may create more discomfort than comfort in the near term, medium or even in the long term. Learned behaviours that have served people well will not evaporate instantly. For some, sharing knowledge will never be as desirable as hoarding knowledge.

As individuals, we have our own calculus for determining the extent we are comfortable with working with others. Technology improvements will facilitate the velocity at which we share information, but human behaviour will at least for the moment determine what we share and how we work together.

In Dan Burke's assessment as Director General, Corporate Learning Programs, for the Canadian Centre for Management Development, the recipe for culture change is not complicated. Leadership, vision and living the change that we wish to see in organisations are essential ingredients. It does not require heroism, but it does entail commitment, action and perseverance. Most change initiatives fail according to Burke, not because of inherent flaws or lack of strategic planning, they fail because people give up.

In any environment, there will be some that will respond naturally or automatically to change. Others will require constant messaging and incentives and inducements to modify their behaviours.

At the heart of real change, as the research discussed here has established, is authenticity and the commitment for sustained behaviour changes. Halfway, 'half-baked' commitments will only breed distrust.

Changing the way people interact and share knowledge ultimately pivots on the key issue of trust. Unless there is reciprocity and trust, at the very best, knowledge management will never be more than a superficial graft, instead of the powerful catalyst for enormously positive culture and organisational change that it can and should be. At the very worst, introducing a coercive approach to knowledge management without a solid foundation of trust can undermine goodwill, knowledge and creativity, to the detriment of individuals and the organisation.

Getting people to do the right thing for some means allowing them to live their values. For others it means changing their values. For a third group it means keeping their values intact, but changing the way they act. Does it ultimately make a difference if people are motivated to do the right thing for the right reasons or the wrong reasons? It is difficult to really know, but on balance, probably not.

While (innate) human nature is unlikely to be mutable, you can motivate people to act differently and shaping desired behaviours begins early, probably long before people enter the world of work. In the words of Dr Alex Himelfarb, 'culture change will happen anyway, if people do the right thing'. In so doing, we will have the opportunity to create a different style of working and learning where, with all due apologies to Sir Francis Bacon, people in the third millennium actually behave differently, guided by the understanding that shared knowledge is power.

Since this research was collected, there have been several new initiatives that have been announced that are creating excitement within and outside government regarding modernisation of Canada's public service. A first and most important step is a task force on modernising human resources management in the Public Service of Canada. The lead minister for the modernisation task force is Minister Robillard, the minister also responsible for the Treasury Board of Canada Secretariat. The task force is being led by a seasoned public servant Ranald Quail, who will suggest reforms based on some guiding principles, based on the values of the public service.

As the clerk of Privy Council outlined in a 6 June 2001 speech to APEX, the Association of Professional Executives of the Pubic Service of Canada:

> The first and foremost of these principles is the need to uphold merit, non-partisanship and competence in a representative public service.
>
> The second principle is that management has to be responsible for human resources management – with all that the word 'responsible' implies.
>
> The third principle is to place responsibility for human resources at the lowest possible level of management, depending on the circumstances, in each organisation.
>
> And finally, the fourth principle is to ensure that managers are accountable for their management of human resources.

The Clerk has confirmed that the new bill should be tabled in the summer of 2002. If successful, these reforms in the human resources sphere may create new momentum to look closely at other ways that government can adjust to prevailing cultural pressures to be more responsive and adaptive to citizens.

Contributors to the research

The author wishes to thank all those who gave so willingly of their time to support this project. In addition she would also wish to acknowledge the high levels of support and encouragement provided by her family.

> Ms Denise Amyot, Director General Recruitment, Public Service Commission of Canada.
>
> Ms Gini Bethell, management consultant, former Chief Information Officer (CIO) Natural Resources Canada.
>
> Mme Jocelyn Bourgon, President Canadian Centre for Management Development.
>
> Mr Dan Burke, Director General, Corporate Learning Programs, Canadian Centre for Management Development.
>
> Ms Michelle d'Auray, Chief Information Officer, Treasury Board of Canada Secretariat.
>
> Dr Marguerite Dove, Cultural Attaché, Unites States State Department.
>
> Dr Alexander Himelfarb, Deputy Minister of Canadian Heritage.
>
> Ms Eva Kmeicic, Deputy Commissioner, Royal Canadian Mounted Police.

Mr Arthur Kroeger, Chancellor, Carleton University.

Ms Jill Larose, Director General, Policy Public Service Commission.

Ms Evelyn Levine, Director General, Corporate Services, National Library and Archives of Canada.

Ms Lynn MacFarlane, Associate Chief Human Resources Officer, Treasury Board of Canada Secretariat.

Mr Richard Neville, Deputy Comptroller General, Treasury Board of Canada Secretariat.

Mr Alan Nymark, Deputy Minister, Environment Canada.

Ms Carole Swan, Associate Deputy Minister, Treasury Board of Canada Secretariat.

Dr Richard Van Loon, President, Carleton University.

Dr Debra Wallace, Faculty of Information Science, University of Toronto.

Dr Aidah Warah, psychologist, organisational development specialist, National Research Council.

Ms Sheelagh Whittaker, former CEO, EDS Canada, EDS Australia.

Dr David Zussman, President, Public Policy Forum.

Bibliography

Davenport, T. H. and Prusak, L. (1998) *Working Knowledge, How Organizations Manage What They Know,* Boston, MA: Harvard Business School Press.

Fulmer, W. E. (2000) *Shaping the Adaptive Organization, Landscapes, Learning and Leadership in Volatile Times,* New York: Amacom.

Goldsmith, M. and Beckhard, R. (1996) *The Leader of the Future,* San Francisco: Jossey-Bass.

Harris, P. R. (1998) *The New Work Culture,* Amherst, MA: HRD Press.

Pottruck, D. S. and Pearce, T. (2000) *Clicks and Mortar, Passion Driven Growth in an internet-Driven World,* San Francisco: Jossey-Bass.

Robinson Hickman, G. (1998) *Leading Organizations, Perspectives for a New Era,* Oakland: Sage Publications.

Senge, P. (1999) *The Dance of Change, The Challenges to Sustaining Momentum in Learning Organizations,* New York: Doubleday.

Chapter 7

Vision and leadership in the digital economy

Mary Harney

Introduction

The remarkable turnaround in the performance of the Irish economy over the past decade or so did not happen simply by accident or because of good luck. Certainly, fortune, as always, had a part in both the timing of events and in some of the decisions made. But decisions were made and risks – calculated risks – were taken. No amount of good fortune could have achieved what has been achieved without the willingness and the capacity to make decisions and to act. The foundations of the Irish economic success story lie in the way in which successive governments and the state agencies developed the capacity to analyse problems and formulate responses, and the way in which they responded to new challenges as they were identified. This chapter shows how this has been done in Ireland and the central role that has been played by key actors and individuals at crucial points in providing the vision and direction that is required to achieve a co-ordinated response.

The programme of action by the Irish government to transform the economy in preparation for a leading role in the global digital trading environment was preceded by a period of intensive examination of Ireland's situation – its strengths, weaknesses and opportunities – and widespread consultation with participants in both the public and the private sectors. The outcome of this consultation was a comprehensive and co-ordinated programme of initiatives. It would have been difficult, if not impossible, for any government to control or even predict how economic agents would react to such changed circumstances. Any attempt by the state to try to control or overly direct the response of the private sector would be likely to fail. The strength of the Irish system has been the ability to monitor the impact that initiatives are having and to adapt policy in response.

Overview of the Irish experience

Ireland is an integral part of the European Union (EU) – a single market of some 370 million people. It is also the only English-speaking country among the eleven founder members of EMU. At the establishment of EMU in January 1999, Ireland ranked in the top three countries in meeting the entry criteria relating to low inflation, stable currency exchange rates, internationally competitive long-term interest rates and a low and stable government budgetary deficit. In fact, Ireland is one of the few EU countries that have consistently achieved government budgetary surpluses in recent years. Current projections indicate that fiscal surpluses will be maintained into the foreseeable future (Figure 7.1).

This position as an economic role model for what can be achieved by a small economy is recently acquired. The fact is that Ireland's economy has been transformed in little more than a decade, from an economy heading for serious trouble in the mid- to late-1980s, to 'Europe's shining light'. In 1988, *The Economist* had predicted that Ireland was likely to remain 'the poorest of the rich' (*The Economist* 1988). There did not appear to be good reasons at the time to conclude otherwise. Little over 10 years later, the OECD could describe our performance as 'the envy of countries around the world' (OECD 1999: 24). In fact, the OECD went further, pointing out that not only had the outstanding problems been addressed but that today Ireland is a world leader in a number of aspects of economic performance (OECD 1999: 25).

This admirable performance has been facilitated by rapid economic growth. As shown in Figure 7.1, Ireland has achieved rates of economic growth over the past 10 years that are well ahead of OECD norms and are actually higher than any other OECD country.

This exceptional rate of growth has been reflected in equally impressive rates of employment growth in the last few years. These have been significantly higher than for the EU or the OECD on average and have also exceeded employment growth rates in the UK and the United States. The extent of this out-performance is shown in Figure 7.2.

Over the most recent 5-year period to the end of 1998, employment growth in Ireland has accelerated to an average annual rate of increase of

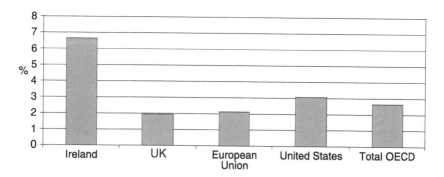

Figure 7.1   Average annual change in GDP 1989–1999.

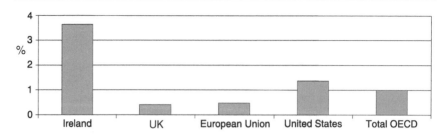

Figure 7.2 Average annual employment change 1989–1999.

over 4.75 per cent per year. Current indications are that significant employment growth is set to continue over the next 5 years.

Unusually, by reference to most other OECD countries, employment in the manufacturing sector in Ireland, underpinned by strong productivity growth, has shown substantive increases over the past 10 years with a significant acceleration in performance over the most recent 5-year period. This is shown in Figure 7.3. Much of this growth has been in modern, high technology sectors which have been a key focus of industrial development efforts as outlined below. However, the service sector remains the main source of increase with employment growing by 58 per cent (392,000 jobs) in the 8 years to mid-2000.

Ireland is one of the most trade-dependent economies in the world. Exports of goods and services from Ireland accounted for over 96 per cent of GDP in 1999, while imports amounted to 82 per cent of GDP. The average annual increase in the volume of exports in the 10 years to the end of 1999 was over 14.1 per cent, while the balance of trade in favour of exports has exceeded 10 per cent of GNP each year in recent years. This performance is primarily driven by exports from high-tech sectors such as

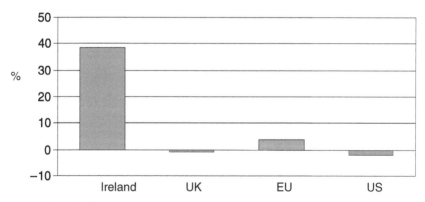

Figure 7.3 Manufacturing employment change 1990–1997.

electronics, software, chemicals and pharmaceuticals. Exports from these four sectors account for over 75 per cent of total exports. This fact alone gives an indication of the importance of FDI to the Irish economy.

The role of direct foreign investment

In the manufacturing sector there are a total of 900 foreign-owned companies operating in Ireland. These account for an employment total of 120,000, some two-thirds of total manufacturing output and over 80 per cent of manufacturing exports. The foreign-owned sector has been expanding rapidly in recent years, in both the manufacturing and the internationally trading services sectors and is particularly strong in electronics, teleservices, software, financial services, chemicals, healthcare and pharmaceuticals.

On a per-capita basis (i.e. taking relative population sizes into account), Ireland is by far the most successful country in Europe in attracting foreign investment. This is the case for investment in both the manufacturing and services sectors. For certain niche areas of FDI investment Ireland is the absolute market leader – irrespective of size. With a population of 3.7 million, accounting for just 1 per cent of the population of the EU, Ireland's market share of FDI projects in manufacturing, software, teleservices and shared services projects amounted to 23 per cent of the total in Europe in 1997. This is more than twenty times its population share.

The FDI projects that Ireland's attractions are concentrated in the knowledge-intensive, high-growth, high-value-added sectors. In the general manufacturing sector, Ireland's market share of FDI in Europe has consistently remained at some 13 per cent of the total. However, in the more knowledge-based and IT-intensive sectors, Ireland's market-share of FDI is significantly higher. For example, Ireland is the absolute European market leader in pharmaceutical/healthcare FDI projects, while for FDI projects in the electronics sector, Ireland's market share is second only to the UK in Europe and the gap has been closing.

FDI in the computer software sector has also been increasing in importance in recent years. Ireland has the largest absolute market share in this sector with some 55 per cent of FDI software projects in Europe locating in Ireland in 1997. This was more than twice the market share of the next most successful country (France at 21 per cent) and considerably higher than the third most successful country (UK). A feature of FDI projects in the software sector in Ireland is that almost 90 per cent of these projects engage in R&D activities. In doing so they draw on a highly skilled work force available to the sector. Similarly, Ireland's market share of FDI projects in teleservices in Europe (over 28 per cent on average over the 1994–1997 period) and in shared services including back-office activities (37 per cent on average over the 1996–1997 period), is the highest in Europe.

The policy approach

The trade-dependence of Ireland's economy drives the public policy agenda in Ireland to a considerable extent. As a country, Ireland is highly supportive of an open-trading international protocol framework that promotes, encourages and facilitates trade between countries. For that reason it operates a non-restrictive regulatory framework in respect of capital flows, an extensive range of trade-facilitating and investment- supporting double-taxation agreements with other countries and a well-developed and competitive financial services industry that is also trade-supporting. A high priority is also accorded in the public policy arena to the development of an internationally competitive logistics sector – encompassing infrastructure, service-level and the incorporation of service-enhancing and productivity-increasing information technology innovations within the sector. Some of the key sectors and key investors are noted in Table 7.1.

The general framework for this policy was put in place when Ireland abandoned an – initially necessary, but ultimately disastrous, protectionist stance. In doing so it moved right across the spectrum and concentrated on foreign industry to the extent that some reports criticised the emphasis on foreign industry as being detrimental to balanced development (*The Economist* 1988). However, the commitment to this policy was maintained. Within this consistent framework there have been a number of reforms in response to requirements. In the early 1980s, a fundamental rethink of the approach prompted a shift of emphasis away from labour-intensive industry towards sectors where long-term growth appeared possible, and a greater emphasis on the availability of a skilled and flexible workforce as distinct from the incentives package. This meant that a limited number of high

Table 7.1 FDI in Ireland: key sectors and key investors

Electronics and engineering	Pharmaceuticals and healthcare	International services	Financial services
Intel	Eli Lilly	Microsoft	Bank of America
Dell	Merck	Citibank	Chemical Bank
IBM	Sandoz	Lotus	Merrill Lynch
Nortel	Pfizer	EDS	ABN AMRO
Motorola	Schering Plough	ORACLE	Bankers Trust
Hewlett-Packard	Bausch and Lomb	UPS	Chase Manhattan
Xerox	Baxter	Korean Airlines	Deutsche Bank
Analog Devices	CR Bard	Best Western	IBM
Lucent	Procter Gamble	Whirlpool	AIG
Ericsson	Wyeth Medica	Cigna	Morgan Grenfell
NEC	Coca Cola	New York Life	Andersen
Siemens	Braun	McGraw Hill	

technology sectors was targeted. The benefits of this strategy would clearly be long term as Irish industry moved up the value chain and it specialised in the sectors that had the best chance of long-term growth.

Electronics and software

The information technology (IT) sector has been a major contributor to the development of Ireland's economy and this has been the case for many years. More than 20 years ago, government industrial policy identified the electronics industry as an industry of major growth potential for Ireland. A number of initiatives were undertaken by the Government to exploit this opportunity. A world-wide intelligence gathering system for key developments in the electronics industry was put in place by the main FDI promotion agency, IDA Ireland. The promotional programme was continually up-dated in response to the changing locational needs of firms to attract investment from the best and most advanced electronics companies in the world. The capacity of the third-level education sector to provide graduates in electronic engineering and computer science was also enhanced considerably. As a consequence, the per capita output of graduates with qualifications in computer science and engineering in Ireland is now among the highest in the world. New research programmes in electronics were developed in the third-level education sector to match the increased resources put into teaching. Crucially, the telecommunications system was radically upgraded in the early 1980s and Ireland was among the first countries in Europe to achieve a largely digitised telecommunications system.

The results from these initiatives are impressive:

- In 1988, the number employed in foreign-owned electronics companies in Ireland amounted to less than 10,000 people. Today the number is over 43,000 people and growing rapidly.
- Nineteen of the top 25 computer companies in the world now have manufacturing operations in Ireland.
- Electronics accounts for over one-third of exports from Ireland. Ireland is the biggest exporter of software products in the world, ahead of the United States. Over 40 per cent of the packaged software and 60 per cent of the business application software sold in Europe is produced in Ireland, while almost one-third of the PCs sold in Europe are manufactured in Ireland.

Considerable government promotional effort has gone into ensuring a good fit between the requirements of foreign-owned electronics firms in Ireland and the long term development needs of Ireland's economy. Today, some 70 per cent of the expansion of the electronics sector in Ireland comes from the expansion of existing foreign-owned firms as distinct from new entrants. These firms are increasingly well anchored in the economy and are undertaking R&D and marketing, as well as promotion activities. Meanwhile, 'new blood' higher up the industry value-chain continues to be introduced to ensure the industry retains a competitive edge.

The electronics sector in Ireland has been evolving rapidly from less sophisticated assembly operations to complex, integrated, manufacturing and software operations, including high-value R&D and marketing functions. Pure manufacturing and assembly operations are increasingly being hived off to low labour-cost countries. In line with these developments, company size is increasing. For example, out of over 300 foreign-owned electronics companies ten companies, now employ more than 1,000 employees.

The electronics industry in Ireland is, thus, an increasingly highly skilled sector. On average, third-level graduates account for some two-thirds of employees in the large-scale projects which companies such as Dell, Intel, Hewlett-Packard, Tellabs and IBM have established in Ireland. Irish-owned electronics companies have also grown strongly in parallel with the FDI sector. They provide a high-proportion of the hardware components and software required by the FDI sector and many are significant international trading companies in their own right. This provides an important strategic balance in the development of the electronics sector in Ireland.

Financial services

Closely related to the underlying factors which have driven the development of the IT sector, the international financial services sector – an IT-dependent sector – has shown remarkable growth in Ireland over the past 10 years. Ireland's International Financial Services Centre (IFSC) is located in the centre of Dublin. It has grown in a few years to become, after Luxembourg, the second largest offshore financial centre in Europe. Thirteen of the twenty-five largest banks in the world now operate from the centre. As of mid-1998, the total of non-domestic mutual funds assets under management at the centre amounted to over €110 billion (Euros) or US $121 billion. In the year to July 1998, the IFSC funds sector increased by 49.5 per cent – the largest increase of any major offshore centre in the world.

There are a number of reasons underlying the success of Ireland's economic policies in recent years. The early identification some twenty-five years ago of the potential of the IT sector as a powerful instrument of employment and wealth creation in the Irish economy was a critical first step. However, the development of a consistent set of government policies over more than a quarter of a century to facilitate the exploitation of FDI investment in the IT sector in Ireland has also been central to the success achieved. These policies were not dirigiste in nature. Rather they were sufficiently flexible to create a business environment for internationally trading firms in Ireland within which a fast-changing global industry could thrive.

Maintaining a competitive cost base in Ireland has also been crucial. Driven by high productivity growth, unit labour costs in Ireland fell over the period 1987 to 1998, in contrast to significant increases in other European countries. As Figure 7.4 shows, total hourly compensation in Ireland is low by international standards.

The relatively low cost-base in Ireland, combined with high productivity rates, particularly in the FDI sector, has translated into high rates of return on investment thus creating a virtuous circle, which attracts further investment. The US Department of Commerce data show consistently that US firms achieve a higher return on investment in Ireland that in any other European country. The data show that in the period 1991 to 1996, the return in Ireland was 24 per cent. Belgium (15 per cent) was next highest, followed by Germany (13 per cent), Spain (12 per cent), France (9 per cent) and the UK at (7 per cent). The attractiveness of these returns are underscored by a corporation tax rate that is among the most competitive in the world. At present the rate of corporation tax for manufacturing and IFSC companies is 10 per cent. As shown in Figure 7.5, this is by far the lowest rate in Europe. A new uniform rate of corporation tax of 12.5 per cent, agreed with the European Union, will be introduced for all sectors in Ireland to apply from 1 January 2003. The standard rate of corporation tax will be reduced progressively to this rate and the legislation providing for this has already been enacted.

These features are important, but the fundamental determinant of Ireland's success in FDI and in the management of its economy has been in the quality of its human resource base. Successive surveys of FDI 'clients' in Ireland indicate that the flexibility and quality of the work-force is one of the areas where Ireland has a major competitive advantage over other European countries seeking to attract FDI. The quality of Ireland's human

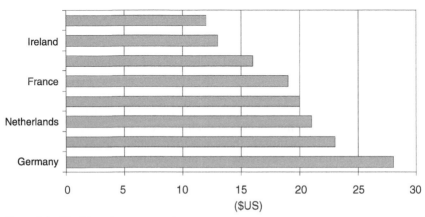

Figure 7.4 Total hourly compensation.

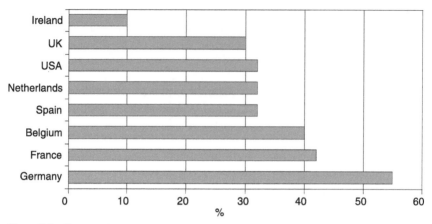

Figure 7.5   Corporation tax rates.

resource base is underpinned by a high-quality education system strongly oriented towards the needs of the business sector. In recent IMD world competitiveness reports, Ireland has been ranked among the best in the world in terms of the success of its educational system in meeting the needs of a competitive economy, ahead of countries such as the Netherlands, Belgium, USA, Germany, Spain, France and the UK.

Social partnership

These strengths have been developed and nurtured over a prolonged period of time, but the recent out-performance of the economy has caught almost all observers by surprise. The real question relates to why performance had been so poor previously. During the 1980s, it was frequently observed that Ireland was exporting highly and expensively educated young people because of a lack of opportunities at home. Irish industrial policy did not change fundamentally in the 1990s, but retained many of the elements that had been developed in previous decades. Certainly there were important innovations, but consistency is one of the clearest aspects of industrial policy.

An important lesson from the Irish experience is that macroeconomic performance has a major impact on the success of industrial development initiatives. Macroeconomic imbalances send powerful negative signals to potential investors. No matter how appealing, on a cost or quality basis, are the resources of the economy, these negative signals are very difficult to overcome. Potential investors view such an economy as high risk and need very good reasons to look beyond this risk. A related insight is that an economy such as Ireland cannot be driven by macroeconomic policy. Macroeconomic performance is better viewed as an outcome, rather than as a target, with performance dictated by the competitiveness of the economy.

Over the years, attention in Ireland has increasingly focused on how micro-economic interventions – such as competition policy, incomes policy, taxation policy and industrial policy – could be used to manage the economy.

Although macroeconomic stability was known to be a prerequisite for sustained and self-replicating development, Ireland continued to experience alternating periods of strong growth and recession, with the recovery always more difficult each time, up to the mid-1980s. In addition, the twin crises of unemployment and debt continued to deepen. Why should each new dawning of economic growth in Ireland be destined to fail, given the country's obvious competitive advantages of being an English-speaking member of the EC with an educated workforce, cost advantages over the other members, a very open policy stance in relation to foreign trade and investment and a highly rated investment promotion institution such as the IDA?

The National Economic and Social Council (NESC) recognised these cycles and characterised them as periods of inconsistent claims arising from a lack of appreciation of the inter-dependencies that exist between various sectors of the economy (NESC 1996). The council, which is composed of employers, trade union leaders, senior civil servants in relevant government departments (i.e. the social partners) and other notable individuals, wrote that:

> Overall, there was an insufficient appreciation of the interdependence of the economy – between the public and the private sectors, between the indigenous economy and the international economy, and between the economic and the political . . . Even in periods of strong economic growth – 1960–73 and 1978–79 – inconsistent claims on Irish output were allowed to develop and were resolved in ways which created major economic problems.
>
> (NESC 1996: 21)

It was clear that traditional growth policies were inadequate. Instead, Ireland required a range of complementary policy initiatives operating within purpose-designed institutions. Many of the prerequisites for this were already in place. The system of social partnership that was created in the late 1980s and operated throughout the 1990s formalised these into a system of co-ordinated consensus policy-making. As shown in Figure 7.6, this had an important effect on the process of policy formation. The key feature of this –

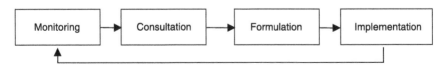

Figure 7.6   The policy-making process under partnership.

highly stylised – figure is the relative positioning of the middle two boxes. In many systems, formulation takes place before a period of consultation. In other words, policy ideas are developed in abstraction from many of the key players on whom their ultimate success depends. In the partnership model as it has developed in Ireland, consultation takes place in structured forums from which either the parameters of policy emerge or recommendations for specific institutions to deal with particular problems are made. The size of the Irish economy and the commitment to consensus means that many of the key personnel that are involved at this stage are also involved in these supporting forums.

There are a number of important benefits arising from this structure. Among these:

- The stances and goals of the main economic agents in the economy are aired and clarified at an early stage.
- Policy formulation can take place in the knowledge that there will be wide support for initiatives that are likely to improve welfare.
- Having found consensus, the Government can proceed with confidence to implement strategies that may require concessions in the short run for longer-term gains.
- A type of corporate memory develops as key personnel and groupings move between the various institutions. This promotes the consistency that successful economic policy requires.
- The system is flexible and responsive to developments in the economy. Requirements are communicated rapidly through the monitoring functions.

The system was initiated in a period of crisis, but has developed beyond its initial design. Its principal concerns were with achieving macroeconomic balance and cost control, and while these issues are still important, it soon broadened into areas of industrial policy and, in more recent years, into equity and social inclusion. Overcoming unemployment has been a central concern, and now that this previously intractable problem has been eased greatly, concern has shifted to the ways in which Ireland can manage its success and prepare for the next stage of its development.

Clearly, therefore, while the upturn of the 1990s was not predicted and could not have been expected to the extent that it has happened, there were fundamental changes in the environment within which industrial policy was implemented. These were far reaching and, in contrast to what went before, the various elements could work together to reinforce each other. The most important of these changes are summarised in Figure 7.7.

In this period, economic policy took on a new orientation that recognised the limitations of the government's ability to direct the economy, while simultaneously emphasising the importance of centrally agreed objectives.

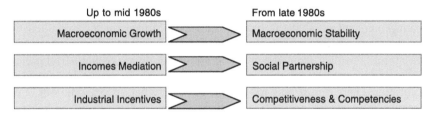

Up to mid 1980s		From late 1980s
Macroeconomic Growth	>	Macroeconomic Stability
Incomes Mediation	>	Social Partnership
Industrial Incentives	>	Competitiveness & Competencies

Figure 7.7   Changes in the orientation of Irish economic policy.

This resulted in a new orientation of policy away from the direct pursuit of economic growth towards creating the environment within which the productive sectors of the economy could prosper. Macroeconomic stability and competitiveness were recognised as the foundations of a strong performance; social partnership was developed as the way to achieve this.

The strategic design of the digital economy

By the early 1990s, a number of the key features, but not the details, of Ireland's approach to developing a leading role as a digital economy were in place. The importance of macroeconomic stability was recognised and consensus had been achieved on how to bring it about. Industrial peace, engendered by social partnership, provided strong positive signals to firms thinking about investing in Ireland. This was aided by a clear commitment to the EU and participation in EMU from the start. But some important deficiencies remained if Ireland was to develop successfully. The issues were identified in terms of three challenges to be overcome in building a leading information-based economy:

- How could Ireland show that it was no longer the poor relation of Europe, but a modern economy capable of hosting the largest and most sophisticated firms in the leading industries?
- How could it capture more of the value that these firms were creating?
- How could it move up the value chain in these industries?

This was a very big agenda and would not occur without a clear strategy. The necessary infrastructure needed to be put in place, preferably even before the businesses that would use the infrastructure were present. This does not just include physical and telecommunications infrastructure, but also the legal and human resources that would be required. In addition, a greater understanding of the factors that give rise to agglomeration economies and the intangible strengths that are required for success in high technology leading sectors was required.

The nature of this agenda and the opportunity to move beyond crisis management meant that the time was right to implement a comprehensive review of the existing policy approach. In 1991, the Minister for Industry Desmond O'Malley, formed a group to conduct a review of industrial policy. The review group, from the outset, stated that there would be no quick solutions. Their report was influential for a number of reasons, not least because it proposed institutional changes designed to ensure a balance between the progressively high-tech, foreign-owned sector and indigenous industry (Culliton 1992). The group did not judge whether or not there was a problem in this regard, but split the agencies into three parts: the IDA for foreign firms, an agency for indigenous enterprise, now Enterprise Ireland, and a new policy organisation, Forfás.

In its recommendations, the group stressed the need to recognise the inter-dependencies of the economy and to implement compatible and mutually reinforcing policy initiatives. Its recommendations covered areas such as taxation, the education system, competition policy, macroeconomics, environmental policy, institutional arrangements and industrial incentives. The group was also influenced by the ideas of leading academics in proposing that Ireland should develop clusters of industries. This was not totally new and reflected the approach that the IDA had been developing, but it drew together in one document many of the strands that comprised Irish development policy thinking at the time. From the vantage point of almost a decade later, and with a transformed economy, the extent to which the recommendations in the Culliton report set the agenda for economic policy in the 1990s is notable. Tax rates have been cut, attention has moved from industrial incentives to providing an environment for value creation through liberalisation and deregulation, Ireland has become increasingly specialised in a relatively small number of leading industries, and indigenous industry has grown up around the FDI core, simultaneously embedding the foreign firms and creating employment in a system of mutual dependence.

Although it was not made explicit in the report, there was also a con-siderable move towards stressing the importance of intangible or intellectual assets in economic development. Today, it is clear that Ireland's greatest strength lies not in its physical assets such as infrastructure, capital or the size of the labour force, but in assets such as the reputation it has created, the inherent intellectual assets of its labour force and policy-making system, the pro-business ethos of government and key economic agents, and the agglomeration economies that have emerged. In a sense this new emphasis was present in the advertising of Ireland of the 1980s that aimed to project a particular image of the country, but in the aftermath of the Culliton report it was realised that this was the direction in which Ireland must move. Being the first mover or the innovator can have important advantages in an information economy. Ireland had not participated in twentieth century mass-industrialisation and it was realised that its future prosperity lay in the newly emerging, knowledge-intensive industries. In addition, the declining reliance on the UK and the emergence of social partnership presented opportunities. It was also clear that there was no single model that could be taken and copied. This belief that Ireland now had an opportunity that it was previously denied was given credence by its success in attracting some of the major players in the new industries. The arrival of Intel is often credited as a watershed given not only its size but also the strong signal this sent that Ireland could support major projects in high-tech sectors.

By the mid-1990s policy began to display a new emphasis on designing the future rather than searching in the present for opportunities. Forfás (1996) provides a key example of this approach. Against a background of strong economic growth – although the old problem of a relatively weak indigenous sector and high unemployment persisted – the report concluded that Ireland could avail itself of some important opportunities provided a long-term strategy to do so was put in place. It emphasised the need for further reform of taxation, greater competition and new infrastructure, and placed considerable emphasis on the importance of education and training. In addition, it emphasised the importance of the service sectors and the role of knowledge intensive activities in deepening competitiveness. In the area of industrial policy, it stressed the importance of new investment in expanded activities by firms already operating in Ireland and the need to pursue higher value-added activity. Thus, the strategy was to both target knowledge-intensive industries and create the type of economy in which they could prosper.

A number of government agencies have been particularly important in realising this strategy. Among these, the roles played by the Information Society Commission and the National Competitiveness Council are particularly notable. The strategy outlined from Information Society Ireland (1996) noted that Ireland was not particularly well prepared to undertake the role it had decided on. Infrastructure was weak as was knowledge among the public of what this new society meant. There were also weaknesses in the use of information technologies in indigenous firms, schools and the public sector. However, obtaining this knowledge was important. The strategy it outlined was built on five pillars:

- Improve awareness of the potential and opportunities offered by the new technologies
- Provide a comprehensive, competitive and low-cost telecommunications infrastructure
- Provide opportunities for learning in formal education and workplaces
- Provide incentives for the uptake of new technologies and concentrate on the development of strong Irish companies in the emerging sectors
- Put in place the necessary legal requirements and public initiatives to facilitate the creation of an inclusive information society.

The need for urgent action to address each of these areas was heightened by a growing awareness of the progress being made by other countries, in particular in encouraging the investment required in advanced telecommunications networks that would underpin all future economic activity in the new economy.

Over the last 3 years, there has been considerable success in meeting the challenges identified above. In a review by Legg Mason, Ireland was ranked among the top four countries in the world in terms of creating a hospitable, high growth environment for the new economy – one of the 'broadband four' along with Canada, the US and the UK (Legg Mason 2000).

Improved competitiveness was a prerequisite for this. There have been many attempts made to measure competitiveness in recent years. The most widely accepted are those that take an eclectic view of the economy pointing to the very many factors that go to determine competitiveness. Conclusions in regard to exactly what these factors are vary, but all efforts point to one strong conclusion in relation to Ireland. Over the past few years, in a period when real incomes have risen rapidly, Ireland has moved from a position of moderate competitiveness internationally to being among the most competitive economies in existence.

The National Competitiveness Council has acted in Ireland to monitor these developments. Firms have long realised that not just costs, but also intangible factors such as design, quality, image and timeliness are important. Similar issues are important at the national level. Partly as a result of its reports, there has been a much greater awareness of the factors that contribute to improving competitiveness. In particular, there is growing realisation of the competitive benefits of a system that efficiently identifies the needs of the people and firms that operate in the economy and that implements measures to address these needs. This more than anything else is the key to understanding the changes that have taken place in Ireland.

Implementing a digital policy and strategy

The IT sector in Ireland is heavily dependent on telecommunications and a good telecom system has been a critical component of the success achieved. Investment in a fully digital system – one of the first in Europe – took place 20 years ago and the system continues to be upgraded to the highest international standards. The telecommunications market in Ireland has also been fully deregulated. The telecommunications regulator actively promotes competition and revised legislation is being brought forward to strengthen the pro-competitive regulatory framework further. Over sixty licences have now been issued in the Irish market since liberalisation in December 1998. While these operators have made substantial investment in new networks and contributed significantly to overall competitiveness, these provide a second benefit by actively marketing Ireland as a location for tele-based activities. Some maintain special overseas offices for this purpose. As a result, the prices available to e-business projects in Ireland are probably the most competitive in Europe. This is demonstrated by the decisions of some of the leading global corporations to locate their e-business centres for Europe, Middle East and Africa (EMEA) in Ireland, such as Microsoft. At present, Ireland also ranks among the most competitive locations in Europe for internet access charges and is the first country in Europe to introduce a reduced-rate internet access charge. All the main population centres in Ireland have widespread cable TV (CATV) penetration and 55 per cent of the population has access to cable services. At present the CATV system is being upgraded to provide widespread access to digital TV, internet access and other interactive services. In Dublin, the CATV penetration rate is 83 per cent – the highest CATV penetration of any city in Europe and for all new building developments CATV access is standard. Cable TV companies are already providing flat-rate internet access charges.

A public-private partnership initiative to provide broadband access to industrial zones throughout the country has been put in place and two digital parks have been opened. One of these parks will provide a base for a cluster of telecom-intensive FDI projects in the IT sector in a low-density, campus environment. The other park will have an inner-city location in the docklands area close to a number of universities. It will focus on the attraction and development of software projects, including multimedia content projects and digital support services. In both cases buildings will be available in advance of demand so that project start-up time can be minimised. The parks will start with a 155 Mbit infrastructure capability, upgrading quickly to 622 Mbits. Also as part of the public/private partnership telecom investment initiative, the government have committed to a $100 million investment project to radically increase international telecom connectivity. Since 1999 alone, Ireland's international connectivity has increased fifteen-fold. The landing of the Global Crossing cable in Ireland, a project initiated by government, connects Ireland directly to the internet backbone and provides direct connections to the US and to thirty-six European cities. The national development plan allocates a further £150 million of investment to regional broadband networks, which should leverage additional investment of over £500 million during the next 3 to 4 years.

Comprehensive e-business legislation has been enacted. The Electronic Commerce Act (2000) makes Ireland one of the first countries to have a transparent and codified legal framework for electronic transactions. The Act creates legal equivalence between traditional paper-based transactions and electronic transactions. This will bring significant benefits by removing all obstacles for e-business transactions and providing a firm legal base on which the internet economy can grow. A business friendly national policy on cryptography and electronic signatures has also been published. Arising from this policy, legislation on electronic signatures and certification authorities has been issued. Taoiseach (Prime Minister) Ahern and US President Clinton, using electronic signatures, co-signed an US–Ireland joint communiqué on electronic commerce in September 1998, which identifies key areas of compatibility in approach and co-operation on e-commerce issues.

Awareness was successfully tackled early on and there have been substantial improvements in the competencies of indigenous enterprises. A number have emerged as global players in sectors that did not exist less than a decade ago.

Just as ICTs are re-engineering businesses they will re-engineer public administrations and the way in which they interface with their clients. Government must give the lead in this regard and pro-actively facilitate the rapid evolution of new administrative structures which are flexible/interdisciplinary and which can draw on a wide range of resources necessary to address the multifaceted issues arising in the knowledge economy – 'form should follow function'.

The e-Commerce Bill is notably an interdepartmental production. This is a best practice example of the way in which public authorities should respond, in a holistic way, to the needs of enterprises and citizens in the information society/knowledge economy. ICTs are forcing companies to re-engineer their business processes/strategies and to adopt new business models. ICTs will have the same impact on government, its offices, departments and agencies. In much the same way as we see convergence in the ICT area, a similar convergence between hitherto discrete government departments and public agencies is necessary.

It is the government's intention to 'e-enable' citizens and businesses – the customers of Government. Essentially, it is envisaged that this will be done by providing a new alternative model of service delivery – the eBroker- which will offer customers a single point of access to services with the potential to eliminate the disparity and duplication inherent in current models. Customers of government will be given the option to do their business, including interactions with the public service, online (through the internet, through PCs, phone, TV, call centres, etc.), whether as citizens or businesses. The objective is to provide online access to fully integrated, customer focused public services. Though processing and service provision will be done by the appropriate agencies, offices or departments, as the customer, will not need to worry about which agencies you need to contact or who needs to do what in those agencies.

There is a world-wide shortage of people with computer-related skills both at the graduate and undergraduate levels. The skills shortage in computer-related disciplines is not simply within the IT sector itself, but is far more widespread because IT applications are pervasive throughout most areas of economic activity. In fact, Ireland has taken the view that, in current circumstances, the over-production of people with IT skills is not possible!

Recognising this, the government established the Business, Education and Training Partnership in late 1997 to assist in the development of national strategies to tackle the issue of skills needs, manpower needs estimation, and education and training for business. The key elements of the partnership are:

- The business education and training partnership forum, which meets twice yearly to consider emerging needs and proposals for action.
- The expert group on future skill needs.
- The management implementation group, which is charged with overseeing the implementation of skills needs recommendations.

In its first report, the expert group focused on the information technology (IT) sector. This report has resulted in significant additional investment by government and the creation of substantially increased places in third-level colleges, at undergraduate and postgraduate level, as well as increased places on relevant vocational and further education training programmes. Provision has been made for a 50 per cent increase in the output of IT specialists from a 1997 base that already provides one of the highest rates of graduate output with IT skills in the world. The increased output will be achieved within 4 years. In 1999, the accelerated technician programmes were expanded to include information technology and 1,100 students are now enrolled on these courses in the Institutes of Technology. The government also approved additional funds for the provision of 5,400 third-level places and 1,500 places on postgraduate conversion courses in IT-related areas. In addition, FÁS, the national training agency undertook to train additional people in relevant IT skills. This additional investment in education and training and the scope of the initiatives in this area has meant that substantial progress has been made in implementing the recommendations of the expert group's first report.

Reflecting this priority, the latest OECD comparative figures show that the proportion of total public expenditure accounted for by education is higher in Ireland than in any other EU country. At present, six out of every ten of Ireland's third-level students major in engineering, science or business studies subjects. There is also a strong ethos of collaboration, between the third-level education sector and companies in Ireland and third-level educational establishments in other countries. These links mean that for most young graduates the transition from academic studies to the workplace is a simple, natural progression. Many young graduates also work abroad following graduation in order to gain experience. The most recent census data show that 50 per cent of the graduates in the 25–29-year age group have spent at least 1 year working overseas, the highest proportion in the EU. Returning graduate emigrants have played an important part in providing the high-level technical and management skills required by the IT sector in Ireland and are an important input into labour force vitality, innovation and enterprise. The FDI sector in Ireland is also largely managed by Irish nationals. This means that there is a large cadre of people with strong experience in the management of multinational enterprises serving global markets available for new investment.

The government recognises that Ireland needs to develop strong research capabilities in the technologies that underpin the development of the knowledge economy. The Irish Council for Science, Technology and Innovation (ICTSI) was established under the direction of Forfás to focus primarily on the public financing of projects in this area. This has also resulted in the Technology Foresight Initiative to identify changes in technology and formulate appropriate responses. This was a major initiative with nine technology task forces and over 160 experts in information and communications, healthcare, and logistics and transport. Following the recommendations of Technology Foresight, the government has approved the establishment of Science Foundation Ireland and a fund of £560 million for basic research in ICT and biotechnology areas. Proposals are also being developed for Ireland to collaborate on research into next generation internet. The government has also approved funding for the establishment of a new research and development institute in partnership with the Massachusetts Institute of Technology (MIT), modelled on the highly successful MediaLab at MIT in the US. The new institute, MediaLab Europe (MLE), will specialise in multimedia, digital content and internet technologies and is expected to attract major international interest and sponsorship. It will lead to new start-up companies and increased entrepreneurship in Ireland.

Setting a new agenda

The environment is changing and Ireland is now at an important crossroads in its development. It is no longer in a catch-up phase, no longer a weak economy that can expect special consideration by the EU. We have succeeded in creating a competitive and attractive economy. Investors in Ireland find a country that believes in the incentive power of taxation, in economic liberalisation and that believes in essential regulation, but not over-regulation. The evidence speaks for itself. Between 1997 and 2000 we have increased the numbers at work by almost 300,000, an increase of over 20 per cent in 36 months. The economy hosts many of the world's leading firms and, increasingly, Irish indigenous firms are emerging as world leaders in their sectors. The economy continues to power ahead on all fronts while there is a durable commitment to a system of policy-making that has been shown to work. Furthermore, its usefulness has expanded beyond the narrow economic concern of a decade ago to embrace solutions to social issues such as inclusion and regional diversity.

This brings new challenges in relation to the handing of economic success for the good of all and the control of expectations. The objectives of

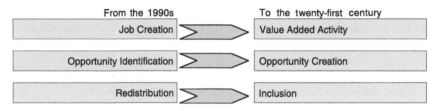

Figure 7.8   The new objectives of Irish policy.

economic policy have changed in response to this new environment, as outlined in Figure 7.8.

This general shift towards quality rather than quantity and towards the better use of resources rather than the use of more resources is evident in the strategy outlined in Forfás (2000). Where previously Ireland could offer a plentiful labour force, it is now facing constraints. Thus, incomes will only grow if there is an increase in productivity. This means that Ireland must not only move into the high-tech, high value-added sectors, but it must also move up the value chain within these sectors. This means that the structural changes that were evident in earlier years will continue, and that lifelong learning will become a basic requirement of the workforce. In addition, Ireland must also ensure that the higher specification infrastructure requirements of this new industry are met.

Nowhere is change more evident than in the IT sector that has played such a crucial role in Ireland's success. Rapid and accelerating technological change continues to shape its evolution. Major discontinuities in trends are emerging. In particular five significant discontinuities can be discerned:

- The technological convergence of the telecoms and datacoms industries
- The major growth potential of electronic commerce
- The huge growth in mobile telephony
- Significant changes in computer software and computer server architecture
- Pre-packaged, desktop-based software is being replaced by personalised, tailored services delivered over the internet.

The on-going challenge for Ireland is to devise innovative ways in which both the private sector and government can undertake their very different but complementary roles and activities to take account of these discontinuities. While complacency is the ultimate threat to the success of any business venture or government policy, past experience indicates that the fundamental capability to meet this challenge exists in both the business and government sectors in Ireland.

However, Ireland is not a rich country in terms of its asset base or its infrastructure. Weaknesses remain, as consistently pointed out by the National

Competitiveness Council. Government policy has evolved to address these and to protect the competitive gains that have been made. Among the most important issues are:

- A much greater investment of exchequer funds in upgrading infrastructure under the National Development Plan, 2000–2006;
- Continued reform of the tax system to reduce income taxes
- The commitment to reduce all corporation taxes to a single rate of 12.5 per cent by 2003
- A major programme of regional development
- Continuing investment in information society initiatives.

Initiatives under this last point are illustrative of Ireland's evolution from searching for opportunities to exploit to taking a leadership role in creating opportunities. Ireland has set itself a target to become Europe's main hub for e-commerce. It now has the most digitised network in Europe with the aim of being the first country in Europe offering broadband connectivity to every home and office. With the global crossing networks, Ireland will have 20 per cent of the EU's total broadband capacity. This capacity far exceeds the requirement of business at the moment, but with the potential of e-commerce to grow at high rates, Ireland will be in a position to facilitate its growth. Given the benefits of being a first mover in high-tech industries, Ireland will also be well placed to offer US companies with particularly intense communications requirements a place in the EU. The payoff from this strategy is already appearing with recent investments by a number of high profile technology firms.

Many countries are now looking to Ireland to adopt a leadership role in many areas, not just business. The Irish policy-making process described in this chapter has a number of distinctive features and is well prepared for this new role. The focus has clearly been on the needs of industry and, while competitiveness will be protected, this is expanding to ensure the benefits are transmitted to all citizens. Long-term strategies are being developed and implemented against a stable commitment to integration into the global trading system. Strategy is decided following wide consultation and the social partners continue to play a role in monitoring and assessing performance after initiatives have been implemented.

The dawning of the information age has changed the sources of firms' competitive advantage. Intangible assets such as branding and reputation have become more important; intermediaries to sort, process and manage information have achieved an enhanced importance; and firms or groups of firms with sophisticated tacit knowledge embedded in their organisations have gained an advantage. Clearly there would be difficulties with drawing overly close parallels between the drivers of success at the level of the firm and at the national level, but the strategy being pursued by Ireland can be analysed against this background. This shows a government approach that emphasises a shared vision and long-term investment. It emphasises consistency and reliability and the need to ensure that all interested and relevant parties are included in the system. Above all, it understands that gains that are built on short-term initiatives, such as public consumption are unsustainable.

The picture presented in this chapter is of a policy-making system that is sufficiently flexible to respond to changing circumstances, but is sufficiently consistent in relation to its core policies to ensure that uncertainty in relation to the stance of future governments is minimised. Implementing this on a national level requires a high degree of awareness on the part of government, an ability to communicate with the citizens of the country and a shared commitment to achieve objectives. Irish policy has a very strong record in identifying emerging trends and shaping the business environment to meet the needs of business in a rapidly changing environment. Recent experience means that this has become even more difficult and more important as the previous challenge of overcoming failure is replaced by the challenge of managing success for the benefit of all citizens. Failure at this time would not only undermine the sustainability of what is in place, but would also devalue what has been achieved.

Bibliography

Culliton Report (1992) *A Time for Change: Industrial Policy for the 1990s.* Dublin: Stationery Office.

Economist Publications (1988) *Economist Country Report, Ireland the Poorest of the Rich, 16* January 1988

Forfás (1996) *Shaping Our Future: A Strategy for Enterprise in Ireland in the 21st Century*, Dublin: Forfás.

Forfás (2000) *Enterprise 2010: A New Strategy for the Promotion of Enterprise in Ireland in the 21st Century*, Dublin: Forfás.

Information Society Ireland (1996) *Strategy for Action*, Dublin: Forfás.

Legg Mason Precursor Research (2000) *The Building Blocks of Growth in the 'New Economy'*, Spring 2000: www.leggmason.com.

National Competitiveness Council (various) *Annual Competitiveness Report*, Dublin: Forfás.

NESC (1996) *Strategy into the 21st Century.* Report No. 99, Dublin: National Economic and Social Council.

OECD (1999) *OECD Economic Surveys: Ireland.* Paris: Organisation for Economic Co-operation and Development.

Telesis (1982) *A Review of Industrial Policy.* Report No. 64, Dublin: National Economic and Social Council.

Chapter 8

E-government, strategic change and organisational capacity

Paul Joyce

Introduction

Leaders in government organisations have been advised to focus on a strategic triad in order to ensure that they achieve the high rate of innovation required for the information age. This entails adding value to services and regulatory activities through the use of information technology (IT), building external support and developing organisational capacity and infrastructure (Harvard Policy Group on Network-Enabled Services and Government 2000). This triad is drawn from a theory of strategic management in government, which has been developed in the United States (Heymann 1987; Moore 1995) and can be used to conceptualise strategic change (Joyce 2000).

The theory serves an important function in opening up new lines of practical action compared with some of the older theories of the public sector. For example, the theory of strategic management emphasises the creation of benefits for the public and business, whereas older theories argued that public sector bureaucrats are unconcerned with consequences because they privilege normatively appropriate behaviour (March and Olsen 1989). Strategic management theory's view that public agencies can and do have the option of forming alliances with other agencies to develop inter-connected strategies (Heymann 1987) might be contrasted with theories of bureaucrats who maximise budgets and over-extend the public services (Niskanen 1971, 1973). Finally, the theory of strategic management takes the view that top managers seek external support for what they are planning and build organisational capacity (values and capabilities) to deliver benefits to the public (Heymann 1987). In contrast the theory of bureau shaping (Dunleavy 1991) assumes bureaucrats shape government organisations to maximise their own utilities (e.g. by outsourcing boring work and creating a non-conflictive environment in their organisations).

The relative utility of the theory of strategic management in government stands a good chance of being tested in practice by the implementation of strategies for Information Age Government, also known as e-government strategies. It is difficult to assess precisely how successful will be the efforts to introduce e-government over the next 5 years and just how functional the strategic triad will be in making it a success. The answer to these questions depends on what public managers are doing now and will do over the next couple of years. Public managers are currently installing infrastructures and identifying opportunities for using information and communication technologies (ICT). Funding and budgeting for e-government has been set up or is being set up. Pilot projects are being set up or are in the pipeline. Recent examples of the use of ICT for management processes, service delivery and democracy may be only partially useful in understanding the introduction of e-government as part of a modernising agenda. This is because they have their origins in conditions different from those now prevailing. For example, e-government in the UK is being implemented within newly established and still evolving strategic and performance management frameworks.

The support of politicians for e-government has been strong and unequivocal. The potential for adding value in terms of benefits to the public and to businesses is generally accepted. This suggests it may be worth paying special attention to one element of e-government innovation: the organisational capacity of the public sector.

Niall Barry, at the Department of Social, Community and Family Affairs in Dublin, considers that building the organisational infrastructure for e-government could take between 12 and 18 months. He thinks that in the first few years there might be one or two clear successes in terms of ICT-enabled public services, and that a continuous process of developing e-government might follow this. However, the course followed by e-government cannot be predicted with total certainty. Even though there is strong political support for e-government innovation, he warns of potential problems.

> The worst case scenario is where the capabilities of the current organisations will be seen to be way too low for what is required, and there will be a mad scurry to buy whatever products out there look the most promising. You will satisfy the need to show visible progress but . . . that will fall away, I would say, in 5 years' time.

Political leadership and support

The implementation of e-government does not merely enjoy the support of top elected politicians. At national level especially, politicians have embraced the challenges of applying ICT to the public sector. The UK's e-government strategy, for example, is positioned as a key aspect of the modernising government agenda.

In the UK, the national government has been the main driver of the e-government agenda. At local government level the top managers are beginning to take the implications of this change on board. They are beginning to think through what this means in terms of the design of services and organisational structures. They are starting to look at how money and assets can be reconfigured to make the change to e-government and presenting their ideas to local elected politicians for their approval and support.

In Ireland, there is a similar political determination to see the Irish public sector implement e-government. Public managers perceive the elected politicians as strong supporters of this agenda. Public managers are well aware of a political willingness to support e-government projects in areas key to the national strategy. They still have to produce good ideas and prepare persuasive arguments for financial support, but there is an expectation that good ideas will be supported financially.

Political expectations on e-government have been made explicit through strategic and performance management systems. For example, challenging targets for e-government have been set in the UK. Public managers are expected to formulate strategic programmes and strategic projects to achieve these targets. The need for challenging targets appears not to be seriously questioned by any public managers. This indicates an acceptance that achieving change is necessary and that public management has a responsibility to respond to pressures placed on them by politicians. This acceptance appears to be in part recognition of some truth in the claims that in the past civil servants and local government officials ignored or even blocked external pressures for change and insulated themselves by conformance to normative behaviour routines, with little regard for the results of government organisations.

Public managers need to be set targets for implementing e-government that are feasible, as well as ambitious. The existence of reporting systems, monitoring and ways of making managers accountable to politicians are essential to make ambitious targets real, but they will only be of use in the face of unrealistic targets if there is dialogue and trust between politicians and managers.

Why are the politicians providing such strong leadership and support to public managers on e-government? One answer is that they can see the rest of the economy changing rapidly and they know that standards of service and responsiveness achieved in the private sector services increasingly define what citizens expect of government services. This is presumably what Pat Collins of REACH, which is a cross-departmental agency established by the Irish Government to develop the framework for e-government, had in mind when he said, 'e-government is out there whether you like it or not. People's expectations are going up.'

Readiness for innovation

There appears to be some optimism that the public sector is ready for facing up to the challenges of e-government. Of course, government organisations are perceived to vary widely in their capacity to change. Some organisations have reputations for being innovative and expect to take the innovation around e-government in their stride. Indeed, there is so much change occurring currently in these organisations that the e-government strategy is being interlaced with other developments. However, not all organisations may have the necessary capacity to respond to e-government.

The approach of national government appears to have been critical in both the UK and Ireland in respect of the readiness of local government to modernise generally. In the UK, certainly for the last few years, there has been an official policy of partnership between the national and local government organisations. And in Ireland a partnership approach has been the hallmark of ICT developments in local government. This appears to have been significantly assisted by the composition and operations of the Local Government Computer Services Board. Brid Carter, director of the board, argues that this has been a factor in the level of understanding among managers:

> The board of this organisation is comprised of seven local authority managers. Additionally two board members from the Department of the Environment, and a board member from the Department of Finance, who is from the technology side of finance. There is a rolling process through which local authority managers get appointed for 2 or maybe 3 years on to the Board here and then somebody else comes on. So over the last 4 or 5 years there has been a gathering pace of understanding by local authority managers of the role ICT can play . . . at this point I would say close to a majority of top level managers in local government are bought in to the whole notion of it, . . . the need to use ICT strategically.

In both the UK and Ireland, there have been champions of e-government. In the UK, during 1999, thirty-six officials and local government representatives became Information Age Government Champions who have a role in winning commitment to e-government across the public sector. Barry Quirk, chief executive of Lewisham Council in London, was nominated as one of two people by the Local Government Association to represent local government interests on the Information Age Champions Group. He has spoken to chief executives and directors of IT in local government about e-government. He considers getting more chief executives personally involved in e-government to be acutely important given the fast-paced changes occurring throughout the economy.

In Ireland, there have also been influential figures in local government management that have set the pace. For example, the Meath county manager, the county manager in Donegal, and the county manager in Kerry, as well as a number of others, have been prominent in the experiments to apply ICT. By their actions, as well as by their words, they have shown their commitment to the vision of local authorities making the best possible use of ICT to increase the effectiveness of management and responsiveness of services.

It is also possible that a major driver for organisational readiness in the public sector is a combination of the effect of many years of budgetary and other pressures and a new policy context for the future of public services. Many public managers would have described the 1980s and the early 1990s as difficult years for public services. But now, the need to invest in public services and, as they put it in the United States, reinvent government has created an environment of opportunities for public sector organisations. Politicians are highly critical of the performance of public services, but they simultaneously value these services. The future looks as stressful as the past for public managers, but there is a sense of challenge rather than threat about the future. The public services have been criticised for being bureaucratic in terms of responsiveness to citizens and service users, but that is changing. Public organisations want to be seen to be doing a good job, want to be seen as innovative, and generally seen as delivering public value through services and regulatory activities.

The question remains, however, have public sector organisations got the managerial and organisational capacity to respond to the challenging opportunities that lie ahead?

The role of the chief executive

The chief executives of government organisations have a critical role to play in recognising and responding to the urgency of the changes needed for the information age. Barry Quirk, chief executive of Lewisham Council in London, recognises that responding to e-government is very difficult. He has tried to promote e-government in local government. When asked for his advice to chief executives on implementing the e-government agenda effectively and swiftly, he suggested that attention was the key.

> I would say that this agenda is central to how you change an organisation and how your organisation relates to the community through service or through politics, through democracy. What do you spend your time attending to? You should spend your time attending to those things that are critical to the future success of how your organisation relates to its public.

Brid Carter, Director of the Local Government Computer Services Board in Dublin, stresses the critical importance of the chief executive for the success of e-government. Their commitment and behaviour has fundamental consequences for the use of ICT. The implication of her views seems to be that the chief executive (and their top management team) has to provide a lead in the move into the information age. Consequently, she places some importance on early attention to management information systems in the development of e-government.

> If the chief executive, himself or herself, buys into it, uses it and keeps it as a high priority, then everything else will fall into place. Champions of e-government have to persuade chief executives of the benefits, and I think they have to provide chief executives with simple to use, highly relevant information. And the only way, in my view, that is easily achieved is through a browser, through a web environment. What they want is relevant information, accessible, easily. Local authorities here that have achieved the most progress, the most commitment, and I think are beginning to see the benefits, are those organisations where the managers will only accept things electronically.

The chief executive has to involve managers and employees in the agenda, generating commitment and also enthusiasm for making use of ICT. This may require the chief executive to go out and personally meet staff and debate with them the importance and urgency of creating new electronic channels for serving the public and responding to its aspirations. At Lewisham Council, they have set up an academy for all their front line staff who have direct contact with the public. The chief executive, Barry Quirk, has spoken to the academy four or five times. He sees its usefulness primarily in terms of updating notions of customer service for new styles of organisations. The council has been encouraging and supporting the generation of ideas for e-government in the operational areas. Barry Quirk is upbeat about this, 'There are more people out there who want to do new things in a different sort of way. And they are different people. They are not like the service innovators of the past.'

Lewisham Council has set up an e-team. This is an informal group from across the council's organisation that functions as a support for the generation of local ideas for exploiting e-government technologies. There is also a high level group of senior managers, chaired by the chief executive and by the director of resources, which is looking corporately at the structure of the organisation and how the focus of technology should be changed.

The chief executive has also to ensure that there is a strategy for e-government. This entails developing a plan, with projects, time-scales and with arrangements for monitoring and ensuring that progress is being made on implementing the plan. The chief executive in local government has also to present the plan to elected politicians and win their support for the necessary organisational changes and realignments of resources and assets. The chief executive, along with the director of finance, has to make sure that this plan is integrated with financial planning so that the budgets are aligned with the needs of e-government.

Managers and experts

It has been argued that it is important that top public managers do not hand over responsibility for e-government to the professional IT experts. ICT is capable of providing a powerful new channel for public services with important implications for the relationship between government and citizens. At a strategic level of management, this may mean that top management teams rather than IT directors should take the lead on drafting corporate e-government strategies for their organisations.

This can be justified on the basis that e-government is but one aspect of the change agenda referred to as reinventing or modernising government. This agenda requires that both the citizen and the service user are the focus of efforts to improve government organisations. It requires organisational and cultural transformations to reconnect to the public (Corrigan and Joyce 2000). In this way e-government is more than a concern to improve the efficiency of processes using ICT.

Some managers feel that IT experts cannot be allowed to control e-government's implementation because they tend to see ICT driving the changes, whereas ICT should be an enabler of modern government. From the IT specialists' point of view there are tensions in how they relate to operational and middle managers in order to advance e-government. At an interpersonal level, the IT specialist can take steps to make their expertise available to managers in a way that seeks to emphasise the importance of adding public value through services and regulation. Niall Barry, who was quoted above, is very sensitive to the issue of how IT specialists support public managers as users of new ICT systems.

> Because you have to assimilate enough of the technology to be able to offer to users education. A lot of the stuff that is coming in e-government originates from within the IT area which reawakens all the tensions between an IT area and the rest of its organisation anyway.

This sensitivity of IT specialists is particularly important where public managers have still to appreciate that e-government could set in train quite dramatic transformations of management, service delivery and democratic processes.

What about the organisational infrastructure for e-government? Some specialists in the ICT field would like to see organisational structures set up that linked together strategic level bodies and implementation teams, and would like to see ICT experts play a clear role in these structures in terms of advice and implementation.

Within the management organisation itself, it is important to recognise the possible dangers to e-government implied by practices highlighted by theories of bureau shaping and theories of mimetic isomorphism (Di Maggio and Powell 1991). These point to problems of top managers relishing intrinsically interesting work of strategising for e-government, while being uninterested in the conflictual elements of achieving a high pace of innovation. This might lead to highly publicised initiatives, but poor follow-though in terms of implementation and then sustaining innovations. Top managers jumping on and off a series of e-government bandwagons as they sought to sustain a reputation for innovation might then compound this. Such a pattern of behaviour by management organisations could look as though strategic management was being applied, but some reality testing might expose the lack of real added value being created through changes to services and regulatory activity.

However, the theories of bureau shaping and mimetic isomorphism are in danger of being overly cynical. A study of information technology innovations in the United States during the early 1990s shows that most are initiated by managers and that innovators work to get staff and clients to accept the new technology, and work to get inter-organisational co-operation (Borins 1998). This same research also showed that while innovations were often comprehensively planned, they were not the result of strategic plans. This could be seen as showing that strategic planning is poor at stimulating IT innovation. More probably it shows that innovation even occurred before there was a strong strategic management framework. Nevertheless, there might be a need to look at how strategic plans can reinforce the drive to innovate and steer the innovations to key areas of the e-government agenda.

Planning, pilots, and project management

One clear message about e-government from public managers and ICT specialists is that it is not simply the application of ICT to public services. It was reiterated a number of times that e-government is the application of ICT in a way that puts the public (or as some put it, the customer) first, and in a way that leads to more holistic or integrated services. Moreover, it was taken for granted that the innovations carried under an e-government agenda would need to be properly located within the new systems for strategic planning and aligned closely with the goals of national government.

The need for a holistic or joined-up approach to public services in part explains the importance of work on the organisational infrastructure for the public services. For some managers and ICT specialists, it was self-evident that this is not easy to achieve if government departments or other agencies work in isolation. The individual departments or agencies need cross-departmental agencies or cross-sector agencies to facilitate the use of e-government for more integrated services. On the other hand, at such an early stage in the modernising of government, experience of partnerships and more integrated services is still accumulating. For the heads of public agencies and organisations there are some challenging questions to be faced concerning the existence of synergies between the activities of partners and whether the search for synergy and partnership working should come at the beginning, middle or end of attempts to introduce e-government. For example, one view is that it is vital to concentrate initially on the interface with the public and the service processes behind it, and only when these are improved using e-government innovations is the time ripe for investigating partnership opportunities through e-government. Of course, this view, which was expressed by a manager, refers primarily to the introduction of e-government in service processes.

Brid Carter, at the Local Government Computer Services Board in Dublin, is concerned with thinking through a sector-wide plan for e-government that can be applied in Irish local authorities. In a way her starting point is the need for partnerships in innovation, as well as in service delivery. She points out that there could be a successful pilot project in a local authority but then it might prove difficult to get the innovation implemented elsewhere. One way of tackling this is to develop a consortium of partners who share an understanding of the desirability and urgency of e-government and for them to collectively launch a series of interrelated projects. Moreover, as these projects are designed and scheduled so that they will cumulatively build into a new model of local government making full-use of ICT, then the projects form a holistic project for e-government in this sector. Probably critical to the success of such a consortium approach is central government support in terms of funding. Obviously, a cost–benefit analysis for any individual local authority to commit itself to be part of a consortium of innovators must be favourably influenced by the chance to benefit from additional investment funds.

In the case of Ireland's local authorities, Brid Carter reports a high level of initiative by individual local authorities, as evidenced by progress made on specific projects already through their own efforts, and substantial interest in taking part in more collective development of e-government projects. The initiatives taken by individual local authorities could prove to be highly important as starting points for more collective efforts. It also seems that there is a relatively high degree of willingness by individual local authorities to share with others.

Thought is being given to how the projects are placed in sequence. First there are projects on core organisational processes such as management intranets. Then, and overlapping with the first type of projects, there will be projects in all of the areas of service delivery. Again, these projects could be building on work already done by individual pioneering local authorities. These projects will involve groups of authorities looking at the way processes of service delivery can be simplified and streamlined, and upgraded to reflect best practice. Then there will be a series of projects that might be seen as more generally concerned with connecting to the public. These might focus on representation, complaints and public consultation. It would seem, then, that the trajectory of e-government, if this plan were adopted, would be to start with the core managerial processes of the organisation and then move through service delivery to processes involving the public and service users.

In summary, the example of Irish local government could provide in a few years' time very important evidence on how well a partnership between national and local government can support a consortium of pioneering local authorities. If it is realised, it will assemble a series of projects into a coherent and integrated programme for transforming the local government sector on the basis of ICT. It is obvious that such an approach offers, potentially, the advantage of mobilising energy for change through its ethos of participation. It is also obvious that the chief executives who lead the pioneering local authorities will carry a major responsibility for sustaining this participation ethos among the partners and for ensuring that the organisational commitments implied in taking part are delivered.

Planning e-government innovations for a single organisation has to weigh up the opportunities for using ICT in respect of quite different processes. Barry Quirk of Lewisham Council emphasises, for example, management processes, operational processes, and democratic processes. E-government can be, and has been, applied to all three processes in organisations in the UK and Ireland.

One approach to identifying specific projects to form the organisational plan is an audit of service managers, an approach that is especially likely in multipurpose local authorities, where there are literally hundreds of services. In such organisations there can, therefore, be hundreds of potential e-government projects. Talking to Adrian Wardle and Julie Johnston, communication specialists in Lewisham Council's Communications Unit, made it clear that the scale of these e-government projects can vary considerably. Some can involve little effort or resources and can offer 'quick wins'. Managers of any programme of change like to get early wins to create momentum and confidence. In the context of demanding national targets required in short-time scales, public managers have to make speedy judgements about what services can go online almost immediately, what services can be offered in the near future, and what changes will require serious process re-engineering. It was also evident that this raises one of those integral tensions of the modernising agenda: combining receptivity to the public with receptivity to national government. Adrian Wardle expressed this in terms of quick wins and usefulness to the public:

> What could be done as a quick win because we want to see progress on the web site, because there is the urgency of meeting government targets for service delivery? [Then there are the questions of] what are the services most critical to get online? What are the services that our customers would actually expect to see and look for on a web site? And what services would the public use most if you made them available? So that process we are still working through.

Inevitably, at the start of a process that might legitimately be called a transformation rather than merely an innovation in the public sector, the configuration of strategic and operational responsibilities for e-government is still emerging. Julie Johnston, also based in the Communications Unit reported, 'My responsibilities are still growing; because it is a new way of delivering services the roles are still metamorphosing.' Julie favours clear internal structures to facilitate getting services online.

It might be useful to register here what might turn out to be an important issue as e-government develops. This is the issue of how outsourcing services and activities through placing contracts with the private and voluntary sectors might impact on the detail and dynamics of the moves to introduce e-government. For example, a public organisation that has outsourced a major activity might decide that its e-government strategy is to be used to influence all activities that it is responsible for, but does this include those it has outsourced, or intends to outsource? If activities are going to be outsourced will management decide that the application of e-government ideas to the activities should be delayed until after a contractor has been obtained? Might management decide that the responsibility for e-government would be dealt with primarily through the specification of the contract? How would an approach to implementing e-government through a contract specification be combined with a commitment to partnership working or more holistic government? Can this be easily handled through the contract or are there peculiar difficulties in this case? With so many e-government projects only just entering the innovation pipeline, these questions can only be raised here.

Greg McDermott was the project manager for the Integrated Title Registration Information System (ITRIS) project, which was a major service development at Land Registry in Ireland between 1995 and July 1999. The conveyancing process carried out by solicitors involves making applications to Land Registry for information in respect of registered titles to land. Before ITRIS was implemented, solicitors sent applications by post and came to the offices and inspected folios manually at the organisation's public counters. Even in cases where technology was being used, it was still a manual process. Hard copies of the documents would be printed out for inspection. Either way, it was quite a costly process for both the customers and the organisation.

From the late 1970s, the organisation had been facing a rising demand for this core service from the legal profession and it was long felt that new technology would be needed to cope with it in the future. An information systems plan in 1990 identified a project in relation to it. The level of applications solicitors were making increased dramatically in the 1990s. In 1994/1995, the organisation started a project to look at the title registration system with a view to providing some technology support giving more direct access to the registers by customers. It was decided in 1996, as a result of analysis, to make the service available through the internet. A new service was implemented successfully by mid-1999. As a result, a manual system of processing solicitors' applications for information was replaced by a web-based system in Dublin and in the west of Ireland. The new system gives solicitors access to raw information of registers of title. They can also create information on the system that produces an online application, and then they can track the progress of their application. As Greg McDermott explains it, by means of the internet the solicitors were in effect brought inside the organisation's own processes. Among the chief benefits of the project's implementation has been faster service for the solicitors and greater efficiency by taking out some of the mundane clerical functions. This allowed the organisation to re-deploy staff resources to other activities.

It is clear from the history of this particular innovation in e-government that making such a major change in a service demanded much effort and detailed work in terms of analysis and implementation over a long period. All staff were briefed, about fifty to sixty members of staff were involved through working groups in the analysis phase, service users were consulted, a case for funding was made to the Department of Finance, and industrial relations issues had to be processed. It was also necessary to change the physical layout of the office, staff had to be encouraged to work in new ways, training was provided, and so on. It is also clear that this innovation was managed within a planned approach. The proposal was considered and approved as part of the strategic planning of the organisation, and project management was used to ensure that implementation was managed effectively and the changes were made within the desired time-scale.

The project management structure used to shape the implementation process was designed to ensure that decision-making and follow-up were effective. There was a project board, a project team, a project manager, and some quality or technical assurance people. The project board reported to the IT steering committee and to the senior management team. In fact, a lot of the people on the project board were also on the IT steering group and members of the senior management team. The project board was structured in this way so that key decision-making could be speedy without the need for referring matters externally.

Greg McDermott, reflecting on the innovation at Land Registry, picked out attention to service delivery processes as being especially critical.

> One of the important things was that we had looked at our internal processes and we had included this idea of external access as part of a process. If you look at any of the interactive web sites where you can do business with it, the process that sits behind that is not the same process that will sit behind a manual application request. Because you are now bringing your customer inside the doors of your office and letting them place information in there, you are actually creating order-processing systems for them.

It was not simply a matter of adding a channel for communication to existing face-to-face and written channels. He considers that process modelling was very important. This involved looking at the process from the request by the customer through to the end when the customer's request for information had been met. Looking at this whole process from the customer perspective also proved important. They spoke to a number of legal practitioners when modelling the organisation's processes and included some of the solicitors' process as part of them. They asked the solicitors what their expectations of the services were and what were their perceptions of how the organisation was performing. For example, the solicitors said that elements of the Land Registry's process added extra work for them. The processing of applications had to be rethought so that it met the ways in which solicitors worked, rather than handling different types of processing separately because that suited the internal organisation of Land Registry. In this respect the work that was done to consult individual solicitors and bodies representing solicitors proved to be very important for the eventual design of the new service processes. Indeed, as Greg McDermott explained, the analysis of processes for the purposes of applying IT can be based on looking at how the public service organisation's processes interact with the customers' processes. He says they try to understand as much as possible about the customers' processes in order to design the organisations'. So it was important that process modelling was informed by the needs of service users.

E-democracy

The Dialogue Project at Lewisham Council began in January 1998 and finished in mid 1999. This project also involved councils in Bologna in Italy and Ronneby in Sweden, and was funded in part by the European Union. It provides another case that might be informative on the realities of e-government.

The project involved recruiting local citizens to participate in an experiment in e-democracy. These were recruited by asking people already involved in Lewisham Council's citizens panel to take part. The participants were consulted on their opinions and these were then fed into council decision-making.

Stella Clarke, the project manager in charge of the Lewisham part of the project, judged the experiment to have been a success, although there had been some technical problems.

> We did manage to consult and people did enjoy using it – even the people who had never used IT before. I think [project management] was essential for the management of the project. Given the short time scales. We are sometimes better and sometimes worse at project planning. There was a lot more emphasis on project management – proper project

management – within the council generally, producing proper project plans.

Stella Clarke also observed that since the Dialogue Project it had felt at times that making progress on e-democracy was facing difficulties because of IT problems, rather than the receptivity of the public. However, in 2000 Guy Rubin of Lewisham Council's Policy and Partnerships Unit has been developing a programme as a result of a paper presented to the council's cabinet, which is the political executive of the council, by the council's e-deputy, who is a member of the cabinet.

> The programme we have developed partly in response to that paper in terms of short-term objectives but also partly more widely informed by the fact that this is an area we were keen to develop. It's an organisational priority – connecting to the opportunities of ICT. So there's a big organisational push there.

Conclusions

Senior managers and ICT specialists in the public sector are seeing e-government as involving much more than simply making greater use of ICT in public services. They are defining e-government as essentially a tool for putting the public first and becoming, as some put it, customer focused. They are also tending to see it as a tool that should be used to assist the public sector move towards more joined-up or integrated government.

They also seem to be assuming that e-government strategies should be developed and implemented in close relationship to other aspects of the modernising government agenda, particularly the strategic and performance management framework. Looking at some recent projects, as we did above, it seems clear that senior managers and senior ICT specialists are committed to making a success of e-government and appear to be championing the implementation of e-government innovations. In this respect we echo the findings of Borins (1998) that public managers, rather than creating obstacles to innovation, are in the forefront of initiatives.

Plans for e-government seem to be shaping up with considerable inputs of strategic thinking, as we saw in the case of the Irish local government sector. We also saw in the ITRIS and the Dialogue Projects that project planning and management is proving extremely useful to managers charged with implementing innovations using ICT. It is even possible, in the light of the remarks of one project manager, that public organisations generally are making more serious use of project planning and management. The managers mention particularly the usefulness of project management in the face of pressures created by short time-scales.

This would seem to be consistent with Borin's (1998) view that rational planning supports innovation in the public sector. However, he found little evidence that strategic planning was important in US public sector innovations. Given the widespread acceptance that e-government innovation should take place within strategic and performance management frameworks, it is possible that e-government innovation will prove to be more strategic than innovation occurring in the early 1990s. Such optimism may turn out to be unwarranted if senior managers do not ensure the integration of strategic plans and e-government strategies.

In the light of the experiences and views of public sector managers we have examined above, it might be concluded that the public sector has become quite an entrepreneurial sector. For example, there appears to be a strong desire to develop the resources and capacity of organisations to deliver more benefits to the public and to do that by bringing together and joining up the activities of different agencies and partners. Indeed, I think the strategic triad does provide a useful guide as to the focus of action on e-government. It is also probably more useful than theories of bureaucrats locked into patterns of normatively appropriate behaviour, or only concerned to maximise budgets and over-extend the public services, or maximise their own utilities.

The strategic triad has to be operationalised in practice. This means managers have to make choices. Should managers go for quick wins or focus on innovations that offer the biggest payoff in terms of adding value for the public? Should decisions about e-government projects be based on a strong conceptual design or should top managers instigate audits of services and activities with a view to assessing each of them individually as a target for e-government investments? Obviously the latter approach might seem more appropriate where there is a large portfolio of very different services, but it should be noted that this might lead to a piecemeal approach that is oblivious to e-government opportunities for synergies between activities. Which types of processes should be prioritised for early attention – internal management processes, service delivery processes, or democratic processes? Should the emphasis be on creating additional electronic channels to supplement existing channels – for example, should effort concentrate on web pages? Or should the emphasis be on re-engineering the processes behind the web pages?

Finally, should spare management attention be concentrated on encouragement and education of staff or should it be concentrated on e-government targets and performance management? Presumably, most managers would agree in principle with the importance of all of these things. However, it is not too implausible to suggest that some managers are happier with an encouraging and educating role, and others happier with a performance management and monitoring role. The former role might be seen as in keeping with the ideas of empowerment and bottom-up innovation. The latter role has been endorsed by the best value policy in the UK. In my view, this might turn out to be a major issue for e-government, going to the heart of managerial conceptions of organisational capacity and how it can be increased. At the present time, it may be important that senior managers are aware of these two different roles and develop management systems that get the best of both.

Acknowledgements

My sincere thanks to the following people in Ireland for helping me with this chapter: Niall Barry, Department of Social, Community and Family Affairs, Colm Butler in the Taoiseach's Office, Brid Carter, Director of Local Government Computer Services Board, Pat Collins, REACH, and Greg McDermott, Land Registry. Likewise, I would like to thank several people at the London Borough of Lewisham: Stella Clarke, Policy and Partnerships, Julie Johnston, Communications Unit, Barry Quirk, Chief Executive, Guy Rubin, Policy and Partnerships, and Adrian Wardle, Communications Unit.

References

Borins, S. (1998) *Innovating with Integrity*, Washington: Georgetown University Press.

Corrigan, P. and Joyce, P. (2000) 'Reconnecting to the public', *Urban Studies* 37: 1771–9.

Di Maggio, P. and Powell, W. (eds). (1991) *The New Institutionalism in Organizational Analysis*, Chicago: Chicago of University Press.

Dunleavy, P. (1991) *Democracy: Bureaucracy and Public Choice*, Hemel Hempstead: Harvester Wheatsheaf.

Harvard Policy Group on Network-Enabled Services and Government (2000) *Eight Imperatives for Leaders in a Networked World*, Cambridge, MA: John F Kennedy School of Government.

Heymann, P.B. (1987) *The Politics of Public Management*, New Haven: Yale University.

Joyce, P. (2000) *Strategy in the Public Sector: A Guide to Effective Change Management*, Chichester: Wiley.

March, J. and Olsen, J. (1989) *Rediscovering Institutions: The Institutional Basis of Politics*, London: Free Press.

Moore, M.H. (1995) *Creating Public Value: Strategic Management in Government*, Cambridge, MA Harvard University Press.

Niskanen, W. (1971) *Bureaucracy and Representative Government*, Chicago: Aldine-Atherton.

Niskanen, W. (1973) *Bureaucracy: Servant or Master?* London: Institute of Economic Affairs.

Chapter 9

Delivering the vision

Where are we going?

Eileen M. Milner

What does this text reveal?

The preceding chapters in this book paint a picture rich in the variety of activities that have been undertaken globally, in support of delivering a vision of public services which are in some way qualitatively different from those that have gone before. Underpinning all of the contributions there emerges a focus upon the imperative for public services to respond to the economic and social implications of the information society and knowledge economy. Essential to successfully achieving this, would appear to be the requirement to maximise the potential for integration across the many layers and tiers of existing models of service delivery. Indeed, whether discussing people or technology, it is clear that all contributors perceive the integration dynamic as being the area where both the greatest potential for, and the greatest resistance to, the achievement of change, chiefly resides. If this diagnosis is correct, then fundamentally, the public service challenge of the early twenty-first century, is to work towards the achievement of services which are seamless from the perspective of the end-user. For this to be achieved, the complexities and legacies of silo-based operation, must be nullified by the emergence of new public service priorities and with them, new organisational cultures and attitudes.

Analysis of the contributions also suggests that technology can only really ever be part of the change story. Far more critical in fact, is the requirement that leadership and vision be in place to both formulate and drive forward a change agenda that is capable of delivering services which actually reflect the lives that people lead and changes within wider society that public services must accommodate. The case studies contained within this text all provide a powerful testament to what can be achieved when such leadership is present.

What is the time-frame for change?

As we have seen, considerable levels of change have already been achieved in some public service domains and it is clear that globally, a powerful change agenda is emerging. However, the migration to new models of public service delivery is ultimately likely to be rather more evolutionary in approach than occurring as a single revolutionary act. The reasons for this are largely related to the sheer scope, scale and complexity of the public service environment and the requirement to fundamentally re-engineer all processes contained within it, in order for profound change to be possible.

However, there is a further reason for acknowledging that the journey to integrated and citizen-focused services is perhaps likely to be longer than some observers are prepared to concede. This is related to the fitness of the user-base (typically the citizen) in respect of their being willing to engage with new modes of service access. Embedding the citizen within the change process represents a critical stage in enacting public service reform and gaining widespread confidence in the new service offerings. Just as public service organisations have to be prepared to critically analyse existing cultures and internal behaviours, they must also acknowledge that the acceptance of change does not occur overnight with a large proportion of citizens. Those who for reasons of exclusion from tools of access, reluctance to engage with such tools or even antipathy towards them, cannot be expected to immediately use innovative information and communications technology mediated public services. To adapt the argument put forward by Peter Drucker in developing his analysis of the emergent economies and societies driven by technological change, change will occur but it is almost certain to take time to reach levels of profound and fundamental change (Went 2000). Thus, the emergence of railways in the nineteenth century was initially a matter of curiousity rather than of obvious economic or social import. This is how we must view many of the changes in public services which have occurred up to now, they are important but we are not absolutely sure, as yet, how important. The next decade will reveal for us whether the parallel with railway development, where potential once unleashed, delivered profound developments around industrialisation and social change, is one which is sustainable in an analysis of the public service environment.

Where do we start? – an argument for turning smallholders into stakeholders

Allied to the over-used rhetoric of the information society and the knowledge economy, is a focus on the term stakeholder, a term which appears to be intended to demonstrate an awareness that all those involved in the delivery and use of public services share an underpinning sense of ownership and responsibility. Interpreted in this way, it is immediately apparent that in an idealised view of public service domains, that a sense of shared responsibility and mutual goals would ensure that aspirations relating to integration and profound re-engineering would be met with some degree of maturity and receptiveness. However, the reality, of course, is often likely to be somewhat different and rather than a culture of stakeholding predominating, the extant model is far more akin to that of smallholding, whereby boundaries and ownership are jealously guarded.

For those tasked with leading public service reform agenda, the need to focus upon transforming smallholders into stakeholders is of paramount importance. Quite simply, the energies devoted to guarding and preserving territorial domains have to be understood and dismantled before significant change can occur. To assume that this can be achieved through restructuring exercises and new organisational charts, is to underestimate the capacity of human assets to impede and sabotage any change agenda. Thus, much of the work around achieving new models of public service has, if it is to be successful, to focus on people at all stages of the service supply chain, to understand their concerns, to engage their commitment, and to involve them in developing improvement-focused service offerings.

Conclusion: where are we going?

Each chapter in this book has served up a perspective on the challenges facing public services as they seek to engage with, and remain relevant within, the emerging, frameworks provided by the information society and knowledge economy. In some contributions there has been evidence of a coherent and credible strategy emerging but of course, it is only through post-implementation evaluation that we can know, with any certainty, whether these approaches have been the correct ones. We cannot actually know the precise direction that public services are going to take, but we do have some sense of the scope and scale of the journey. One thing of which we can be certain, however, is that there is emerging a sense of both urgency and energy around the need to refocus the emphasis and direction of public services. It is this gathering momentum which should ensure that the early decades of the twenty-first century, are likely to be characterised by an emphasis upon articulating credible public service visions; achieving the delivery of change and developing a capacity for revision of developments and of associated cultures.

Reference

Went, R. (ed.) (2000) *Globalization,* Pluto Press: New York.

Index

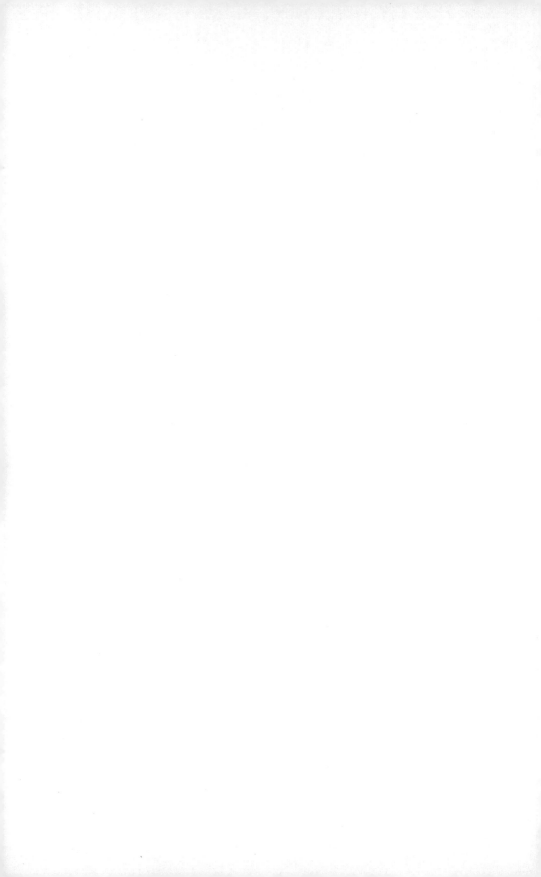